BEE IN BALANCE

10/11/94
~ For Margaret ~
With Love & Best Wishes
Amber

Amber Rose, L.Ac., L.C.S.W.

Starpoint Enterprises, Ltd. ✳
Bethesda, Maryland

This book is not intended to replace the services of a licensed health care provider in the diagnosis or treatment of any illness or disease. Any application of the materials or techniques set forth in this book is at the reader's discretion and is the reader's or their consenting patient's sole responsibility.

Library of Congress Cataloging-in-Publication Data

Rose, Amber

Bee in Balance: A Guide to Healing the Whole Person with Honeybees, Oriental Medicine, & Common Sense; Alan Dumoff, editor.

1. Holistic Medicine 2. Bee Venom Therapy 3. Acupuncture

I. Title

615.89 RO

Illustrations by Shonne N. Farrell, B.F.A.
Desktop Publishing by Alan Dumoff
Forward by Charles Mraz
Introduction and Sting Instructions by Pat Wagner

Grateful acknowledgement is made to the following for permission to reprint previously published material:

"Hope Stings Eternal" reprinted with permission from The Washington Post.

Excerpt from Dianne Connelly, All Sickness is Homesickness. Columbia, MD: The Traditional Acupuncture Institute, 1993, reprinted with permission.

Library of Congress Catalog Card Number: 94-067220
ISBN: 0-9641810-0-2

Cover design by Fishergate, Inc. of Annapolis, Maryland
Cover Calligraphy by Hua Hao

Printed in the United States of America
September 1994

For my son, Reuben Skye Rose

"We have the same heart . . . ❤"

"A LITTLE BIT OF BEES, A LITTLE BIT OF GOD, & A WHOLE LOT OF ME!"

LONNY'S STORY

I got my first symptoms in 1983. My left eye went blind but the doctors had no idea what was wrong. The doctors put me in the hospital. I will never forget this one day when I saw an old man crying because he couldn't see. I remember thinking, "I'm so lucky . . . at least I still have one good eye!" A month later the doctors told me that they thought I had MS. I had no idea what that was. Then several months later I began to have trouble with my right eye. I got to the point that I could only see shadows. On January 11, 1985, I was on my way out of the community center when I realized that I couldn't see anything at all. I was too scared to tell the receptionist that I was blind. I believed in my heart that I could make it home if I could just make it to this one mailbox. I eventually found my way home. I sat there all alone in the dark and cried. I went into a deep depression. I eventually pulled out of it when I got hooked up with The Lighthouse for the Blind. They taught me independent living skills and how to read Braille. Some time later I began to have trouble walking. The doctors gave me steroids, which caused me to develop sugar diabetes. In June 1987, I had another flare up. I couldn't hold my fork, my hands and arms became weak, and I lost all the strength in my legs. I was afraid I would never walk again. I had my ups and downs after that. I was in and out of the hospital for years and eventually I went into a nursing home in August of 1992, at the age of 36.

In September of 1993, I had my first 6 bee stings. I have been feeling better ever since. It has been uphill for me all the way. I have had no bad days. I owe it all to Pat Wagner and Amber Rose. It used to take two nurses to help me transfer from the bed to the wheelchair. After the first few weeks of bee stings it only took one nurse to help me. Then I started wheeling myself around in the chair, because I had more strength in my arms.

My arms and hands have gotten so strong now that I can actually feed myself for the first time in years. I can eat Chinese food all the time now . . . all by myself. I can hold my radio in my hand and change the stations on my own. This makes me feel good about myself. I don't like depending on other people all the time. I like doing things for myself.

On March 20, 1994, I had my miracle. I started to walk again. I have been using the parallel bars and the walker. This is really something! I'm gonna get out of here! People ask how I did it and this is what I tell them, "A little bit of bees, a little bit of God, and a whole lot of me!"

LONNY IS AN INSPIRATION TO US ALL! HE ALWAYS HAS A POSITIVE ATTITUDE AND A SMILE ON HIS FACE. HE MAY BE BLIND, BUT HE HAS SEEN THE LIGHT. ONE DAY I SAW HIM SITTING IN MY LIVING ROOM WAITING FOR HIS RIDE FROM THE RED CROSS. HE WAS SITTING THERE SO QUIETLY THAT I ASKED HIM IF HE WAS BORED. "OH, NO!" HE REPLIED. "I'M JUST THINKING ABOUT ALL THE GOOD THINGS THAT ARE GOING TO HAPPEN TO ME!" A.R.

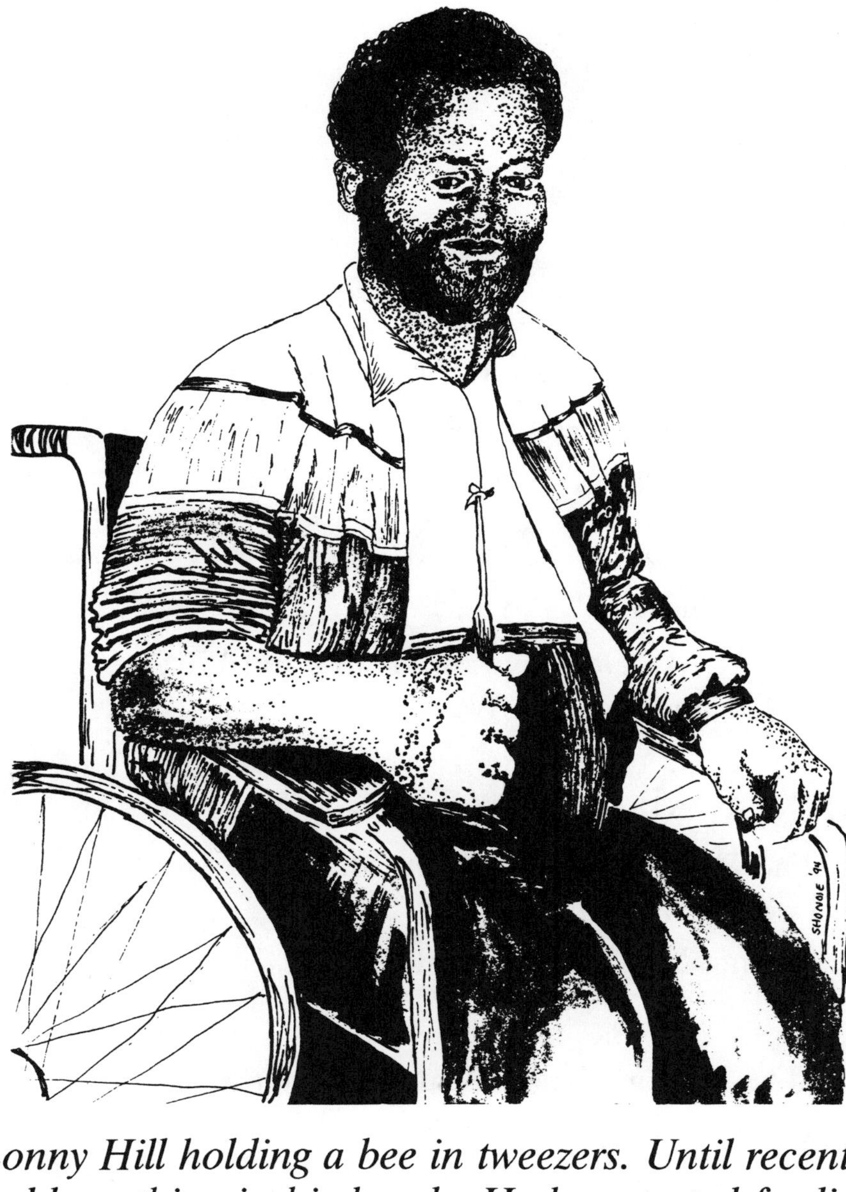

This is Lonny Hill holding a bee in tweezers. Until recently he wasn't able to hold anything in his hands. He has started feeding himself.

TABLE OF CONTENTS

PART 3: COMMON SENSE

APPENDICES

ACKNOWLEDGEMENTS

This book was basically written in three months time, with a self-imposed deadline: the AAS annual conference in the fall of 1994. On the other hand, I have been writing this book or preparing for this book all my life. . . . The typing occurred over a three month period, in the midst of a very busy schedule . . . staying up to 2 a.m. many nights in a row . . . and still getting up at 6:20 a.m. to take my son to school. I learned how to use the computer from scratch while writing this book. I don't usually think that I work well under pressure . . . but my anxiety to meet my deadlines pushed me forward at an uncontrollable frenzy at times. I was as busy as a bee. Staring at my hives for inspiration, I certainly understood what that means! As well as the thousands of honeybees who have contributed to my patients' well-being, I'd like to take the opportunity to thank all the people who kept me going these last few years and those who helped make this book possible.

ON A PERSONAL NOTE:

❧ Reuben Skye Rose, my son—who kept me going all these years . . . who believed in me, who had many dinners alone because I was working late . . . and when we ate together we often had bees, tweezers, spray bottles and computer paper on the table. . .

❧ My student, friend and companion Hubert Duke, who coached me and encouraged me on, who loaned me the computer to write this book, bought a new keyboard when the old one gave out . . . always made sure I ate . . . brought lunches or took me out to dinner after a long day . . . arranged for a woman to come and help me clean my house once a week so I could focus on the book and meet my deadlines. . . . Duke, I could not have written this book without your loving support.

❧ Thanks to George Kalish, my long-time friend and Zen-Master who is forever reminding me, ever so gently, what life is all about and what really matters. Thank you for all the late night phone calls that lasted hours and for seeing through the surface issues down to the core problems. Your enthusiasm was contagious . . . and you reminded me over and over again . . . who I really am and what I came here to do.

❧ Thanks to Myrna Alexander who walked me through my life every step of the way this last year . . . I will always be grateful.

❧ Thanks to Alicia Foster for all her support.

❧ Thanks to Wendie Wheaton, my "adopted" daughter, who was more like a mother to me this year.

❧ And to my sister Beth Rosen . . . who never stopped calling to see how I was these last few years . . . and who forgave me for all the times that I forgot to ask her how she was doing.

❧ And for Alan Dumoff who was always there when I needed his support on every level.

❧ For all my 12-step friends, especially the women in the Tuesday morning meeting, who gave me the courage to go on with my life when I felt discouraged . . . .especially my sponsor, Barbara.

❧ For Kirby Lemesh who believed in me all these years. When I questioned my path he made the statement that changed my life: "Only you can write the next chapter."

❧ For all my friends in St. Mary's County . . . you know who you are . . . who knew me before I found the bees.

❧ For my landlord who didn't kick me out when they found out I had four hives and was stinging people with bees. Thanks echoed by my many patients . .

❧ For the people who rented this house before me . . . and left in such a hurry that they forgot to cancel their subscription to the Washington Post. . . . I got about 6 months of free newspapers . . . most of which I did not read . . . but fortunately read the article about Pat Wagner.

❧ For my neighbors on Roosevelt St. who have never complained about my beekeeping.

❧ For Diane Pilikian who grew her garden this spring in my backyard and shared her produce and her love.

❧ To my mother and father, Lillian and Sidney Rosen, who in their own quiet way were always "rooting for me."

❧ For Heather Stroup, John and Lou Milne, Leo Montgomery and Dave who watched my animals while I was out of town.

❧ Thanks also to those who drove me to the airport for all my trips: Lou Milne, Dave, Art Jaffee, Steve Heflin, and Hubert Duke.

❧ Special thanks to Julie Wilson at the Bank of Baltimore for her TLC. She probably still does not know how much her smile helped. It is really true that one person can make a difference.

NOTEWORTHY "BEE PEOPLE"

❧ Special thanks to Jennifer Fellows who first told me she was having success with the bee stings . . . my fairy godmother who got me into the bees . . . introduced me to Dr. Bruce Rind, who hired me on the spot to work in his clinic. Yes, thank you Jennifer for your smiling face that always keeps me going.

❧ To Pat Wagner, "the Bee Lady," and her husband, "Sting Ray," who let me into their home . . . and taught me everything they knew . . . who gave me a sense of family at a time in my life when I really needed to belong to something . . . who encouraged me to go to China . . . and have encouraged me to explore the connection between BVT and acupuncture.

❧ And for Mickey and Joyce Harwell who were good role models for me in keeping things calm when you have 30-50 people in your living room getting bee stings . . . and especially to Mickey for teaching me how to catch the bees on tweezers without spraying them to death . . . and for giving me the first set of locking tweezers . . . which are so hard to come by.

❧ For Anne-Marie Verstegen who bought me my first hive and watched my progress unfold, and encouraged me every step along the way.

❧ For Marisa and Louis who took over the "sting operation" when I went to China . . . and did a great job.

❧ For Carolyn and Henry Harrell, who often volunteered on their lunch hour. And Rae Carol Tekeste and Olivia Cook who helped when they could.

❧ To the Clark DeFranceaux who built the access ramp to my house on such short notice.

❧ To Mildred Dickenson who paid to have the railing put on the steps so people would feel more confident walking up the stairs.

❧ For Donaldson Welding Co. who built the railing at a reduced price.

❧ For Charlie Mraz who made me feel special and believed in my ideas about combining acupuncture and bee venom therapy . . . who gave me three of his best hives . . . who initiated me into the world of bees on a 13 hour drive from Vermont to Maryland with those hives in the back of the station wagon. The hives opened up and the bees were crawling all over us for hours and neither of us got stung . . . .and who showed me everything he knew about bee venom collection. And special thanks to his daughter Michelle Mraz-Kurker for all her support.

❧ To Kate Chatot, R.N., my China roommate, who will be my sister forever, who reminds me to pick up only my own suitcase . . . and speaking of suitcases . . . to all my China buddies who carried my suitcase (the heaviest one) all those times. To the Pine St. Benevolent Society who encouraged me onward. To Jim Smith who welcomed Charlie and me in Arizona and helped us collect bee venom this winter.

❧ To Bradford Weeks, a principal lecturer in the field . . .

❧ Thanks to Lonny Hill who inspired us all . . . who got up and started walking again after a year and seven months. . . who never gave up . . . and taught me so much about positive attitudes.

❧ To Leo Montgomery for helping me collect 30 jars of bees every week and doing my dishes.

❧ Thanks to all the patients who let me sting them with bees in acupuncture points . . . for practicing "living acupuncture" on them . . . who brought me tissues, toilet paper rolls, jars, index cards, paper towels, etc.

❧ To all the groups that invited me to speak.

❧ For Hubert Duke who was here practically night and day collecting bees, filling jars with honey, putting bees on tweezers and stinging people in nursing homes.

❧ For Frank Shore, the state Senator, who believed in me and called me "the Queen Bee" . . . and is one of my biggest fans and most enthusiastic supporters.

❧ For Greg Ferris for helping me find a way to get bees-by-mail to the people who need them.

❧ For Ernie Muhly who patiently helped me work the hives the first spring and arranged for me to get some good, inexpensive equipment.

❧ For George Imrie who helped me when my bees swarmed . . . and thanks to all the other Montgomery County beekeepers.

❧ To Steve Heflin, the driver of the handicapped taxi, who learned to sting people and continues to do so right in the taxi.

❧ To Joe Hoyle, the volunteer driver, (and all the people from the Montgomery County Red Cross) who arranged for transportation for patients to get their stings twice a week.

As you can see, this has been quite an adventure!

FOR THOSE WHO HELPED DIRECTLY WITH THE BOOK

❧ Comments that made a difference from: Alan Dumoff, Charlie Mraz, Kate Chatot, R.N., Meg Mills, Hubert Duke, Michael Broffman, L.Ac., Michael McCulloch, L.Ac., Theodore Cherbuliez, M.D. and his wife Susan, Lorraine Foxworth, Dr. Peter Martin, Perry Perretz, Diane Pilikian, Alicia Foster, and especially to George Kalish who read the book word by word, like a reading meditation . . . giving me ideas that would change this book and my life forever.

❧ Typing: Judy Silverman and her mother, Marie Glucksberg, Fred Sandberg.

❧ People who taught me how to use the computer: Fred Sandberg, Alan Dumoff, and Kirby Lemesh.

❧ To Alan Dumoff for his excellent ideas as editor, desktop publishing, help with book design and for his legal consultations.

❧ Nutrition chapter . . . Dr. Myrna Alexander.

❧ Shonne N. Farrell, M.B.A., who helped with the artwork at the last minute.

❧ Dr. Bruce Rind, who let me use his xerox and fax machines, and special thanks to his office staff as well.

❧ For Dianne Connelly who allowed me to quote from her book, "All Sickness is Homesickness," in Chapter 6.

❧ Special thanks to Jim Smith for his excellent information on keeping bees alive in a jar.

❧ Thanks also to Professor Harry Gaynor from the National Burn Victim Foundation for his information on the Moist Exposed Burn Ointment (MEBO).

❧ Thanks to Lillian Whitis and the other librarians in the Montgomery Country library for their helpful assistance.

❧ Special thanks to Tom Valeri for his assistance with cataloging in publication.

❧ Thanks to Michael Simics for his encouragement and excellent tips on self-publishing as well as his assistance in providing technical information which you'll find in the appendix.

❧ Thanks to Sally Ehrlich Hoffman for help with the title of the book and for her beautiful photograph which inspired the cover.

❧ Special thanks the staff at the North China Restaurant in Bethesda for the translation of the title into Chinese and for Hua Hao for the calligraphy used in the title.

AND REGARDING ACUPUNCTURE

❧ The staff at Traditional Acupuncture Institute.

❧ Dr. Rind for believing in me and sending me patients.

❧ All my acupuncture patients who taught me more than I could learn from any book.

❧ To all my acupuncture/massage students who always remind me just how much I love teaching.

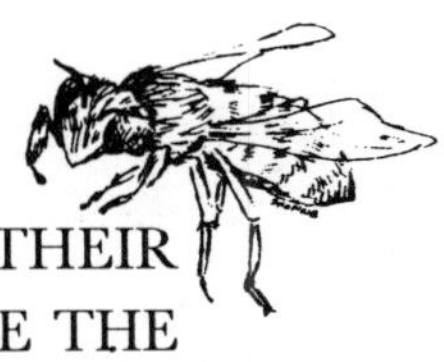

AND MOST OF ALL TO THOSE WONDERFUL HONEYBEES WHO GAVE THEIR LIVES SO SELFLESSLY TO HELP US HEAL OURSELVES. THE HONEYBEES ARE THE ONLY CREATURES ON THE EARTH THAT IMPROVE THE ENVIRONMENT AND DO NOT PREY ON ANY OTHER SPECIES. WE HAVE A LOT TO LEARN FROM THEM.

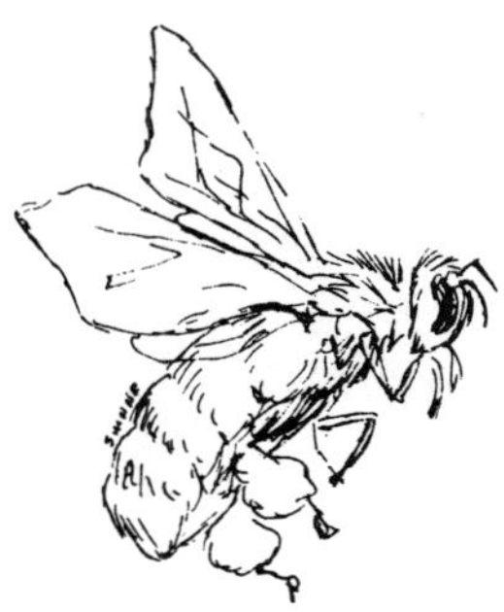

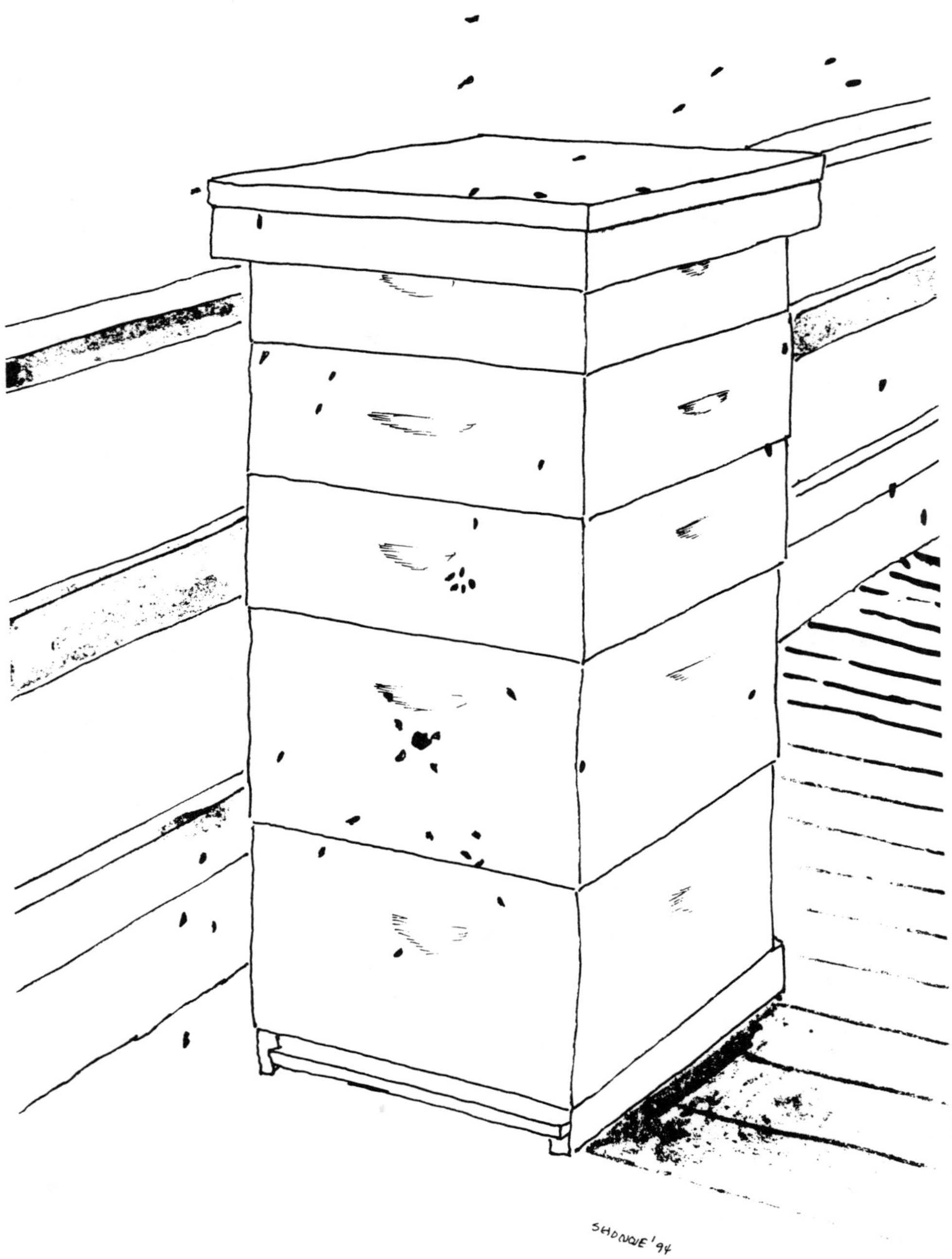

***Bees in Balance**: This is one of the hives on my deck that Charlie Mraz and I brought down from Middlebury, VT. I'll never forget how the hives opened up on that 13 hour drive and the bees were crawling all over me. That was my initiation. I did not get any stings.*

FOREWORD

"A GIFT FROM GOD"
CHARLES MRAZ

For many years, Bee Venom Therapy (BVT), the use of bee stings to treat many forms of Rheumatic Diseases, was known and practiced by very few people. These people usually stumbled upon the "wonder treatment" through some personal experience of their own.

My life-long interest in BVT came as a result of a violent attack of rheumatic fever in early January, 1934. I seem to remember it starting out as a flu or a cold. I was 28 years old and I guess I thought I was indestructible so I kept on going. The rheumatic fever must have started one day when I suddenly passed out on the bathroom floor. After I crawled back into bed, that's when the pain started. First it attacked my back. It felt like my back had just been cleaved by an axe. The next day the pain went to my knee, which felt like it was being smashed by a sledge hammer. The disease attacked a new joint every day. And let me tell you, the pain was unbearable. One night the pain was so intense that I remember wanting to cut my leg off so I could have some relief. Finally after two weeks, I was able to get out of bed again, but I was no longer a young man of 28. My joints were so painful and stiff that I felt more like an old man of 98.

"AS A BEEKEEPER THROUGH THE YEARS, I HAD HEARD ABOUT THE OLD WIVE'S TALE THAT BEE STINGS WERE GOOD FOR ARTHRITIS. I WAS UNCONVINCED. I THOUGHT ARTHRITIS WAS WHAT OLD PEOPLE IMAGINED THEY HAD JUST TO GET SYMPATHY."

As a beekeeper through the years, I had heard about the old wive's tale that bee stings were good for arthritis. I was unconvinced. I thought arthritis was what old people imagined they had just to get sympathy. And the idea of using bee stings for arthritis was utterly ridiculous.

Boy, was I wrong! I guess the "man upstairs" had a big lesson to in store for me. The arthritis nearly crippled me. There were times I couldn't even get out of a chair and my knees were so painful that I had great difficulty walking. Then one day in July of 1934 I got so tired of the pain in my knees that I broke down and decided to sting myself once on each knee in the MOST tender spots. I promptly forgot about it and went on with my day.

The next morning I woke up and I knew something was wrong immediately. "What's wrong with my knees? They don't hurt anymore!" I could hardly believe it. I was in a state of shock. I even started to question my sanity. I wondered if I had really had arthritis for the last six months or if it had just been my imagination.

But here we are, almost sixty years later, and I know without a shadow of a doubt that those two bee stings cured my arthritis overnight. This was a dramatic turning point in my life. From that personal experience, I have treated many people through the years, from July 1934 to the present time, 1994.

> "THE NEXT MORNING I WOKE UP AND I KNEW SOMETHING WAS WRONG IMMEDIATELY. 'WHAT'S WRONG WITH MY KNEES? THEY DON'T HURT ANYMORE!'"

Treating a rheumatic disease, like arthritis, did not create too much interest in the medical profession, as they preferred the easier and more profitable treatment for arthritis with drugs. Some thirty years ago I wanted to try to treat Multiple Sclerosis with BVT. I considered it to be a rheumatic disease and since it had no satisfactory medical treatment, I thought maybe BVT might help. As can be imagined, anyone diagnosed with MS was not going to submit to any "crazy treatment" like bee stings. Bee venom therapists were considered "nuts" with "bees in their bonnets."

It wasn't until 1980 that a lady came to me to treat her arthritis. She was fine for five years, when some of the symptoms returned. She went back to her doctor who told her she did not have arthritis. She had MS! And he told her that she'd had MS for at least six to ten years. She was very upset because her mother had died with MS. She was very aware of what this diagnosis meant for her.

She then came to see me again to tell me that five years before, when I had successfully treated her for "arthritis," I was actually treating her for MS! And she was fine for five years. She decided to come back and try it once more. Again, she made a dramatic recovery after five months of treatment. Though treatments with bee venom have been terminated for seven years, she is still symptom-free.

In my talks on BVT I started to tell people about my success with MS. In contrast to BVT for arthritis, BVT for MS generated an almost instantaneous interest with many victims of MS all over the United States. There was nothing else to help them. Results with BVT on MS has shown improvement in almost all cases treated.

Very few people have serious interest in BVT, since it is difficult to understand and not easy to apply the live bees to the effected areas of MS and arthritis patients. Amber Rose is a professional acupuncturist in Maryland. When she first read about BVT for treating MS, she became instantly interested in the subject. I have known for years that acupuncture and BVT are so closely related. It is a natural thing to apply the bee stings to the many acupuncture points of the body to get the best results.

I first met Amber Rose on a flight from Tokyo to Hong Kong on the way to an apitherapy conference in China in September 1993. She started to talk to me about BVT. Having sixty years experience on the subject, I can usually tell in the first minute or so if the person knows what they are talking about or if they are a phony. I was amazed at her intimate knowledge of the subject. She talked like a professional apitherapist. There are few people in the world who know anything about the subject, so to meet Amber Rose was a wonderful experience.

Amber received her first training in apitherapy working with Pat Wagner, an MS victim who made a dramatic recovery with BVT. When the news of Pat's success reached the media, Pat's home was invaded with crowds of MS patients looking for help. Amber Rose jumped in at Pat's home, volunteering her time and energy to treat those people looking for help.

It is amazing how fast Amber learned to carry out the treatment under Pat Wagner's direction. When Pat took some time off, many of the MS patients started to come to Amber's home. What is incredible to me is that Amber says of all the cases she's treated, only one person has not responded. That's a darn good percentage, 99%!

My experience since I first started treating MS about 1985 has been that most cases do show some improvement. How much varies with each case. We still have a lot to learn about how to treat MS with BVT. What is most important is that it works. In addition, the treatment has no adverse side effects, and bees can be secured from beekeepers at a very low cost. They can even be caught in a jar (with honey in it) in any flower garden for nothing.

A successful treatment for an incurable disease like MS, that has no adverse side effects and costs almost nothing, has to be a gift from God and Mother Nature. We hope more dedicated health practitioners, like Amber Rose, especially those with experience and training in acupuncture, will join in to treat all those who suffer from MS.

Amber has often said to me that she thinks some day I will get the Nobel Prize for my work. But I say, "No, I'm just nothin' but a nothin'." Now Amber, she's somethin' else. She is my Nobel Prize. It is so uplifting, after all this time, that someone like Amber came along, saw the value and the importance of what I have been trying to do for sixty years, and brought it to another level. I know that she will carry on my work long after I am gone. I appreciate her efforts and I am very proud of her accomplishments. I wish her well.

To all of you out there reading these words, please don't give up. Just be patient and give BVT a chance. It is not a magic one-shot pill, it is a means to help the body heal itself.

GOOD LUCK

AND GOD BLESS YOU

Charles Mraz

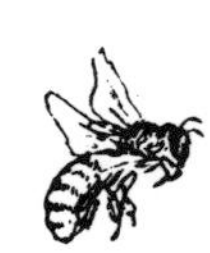

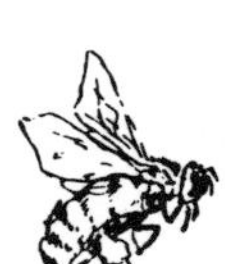

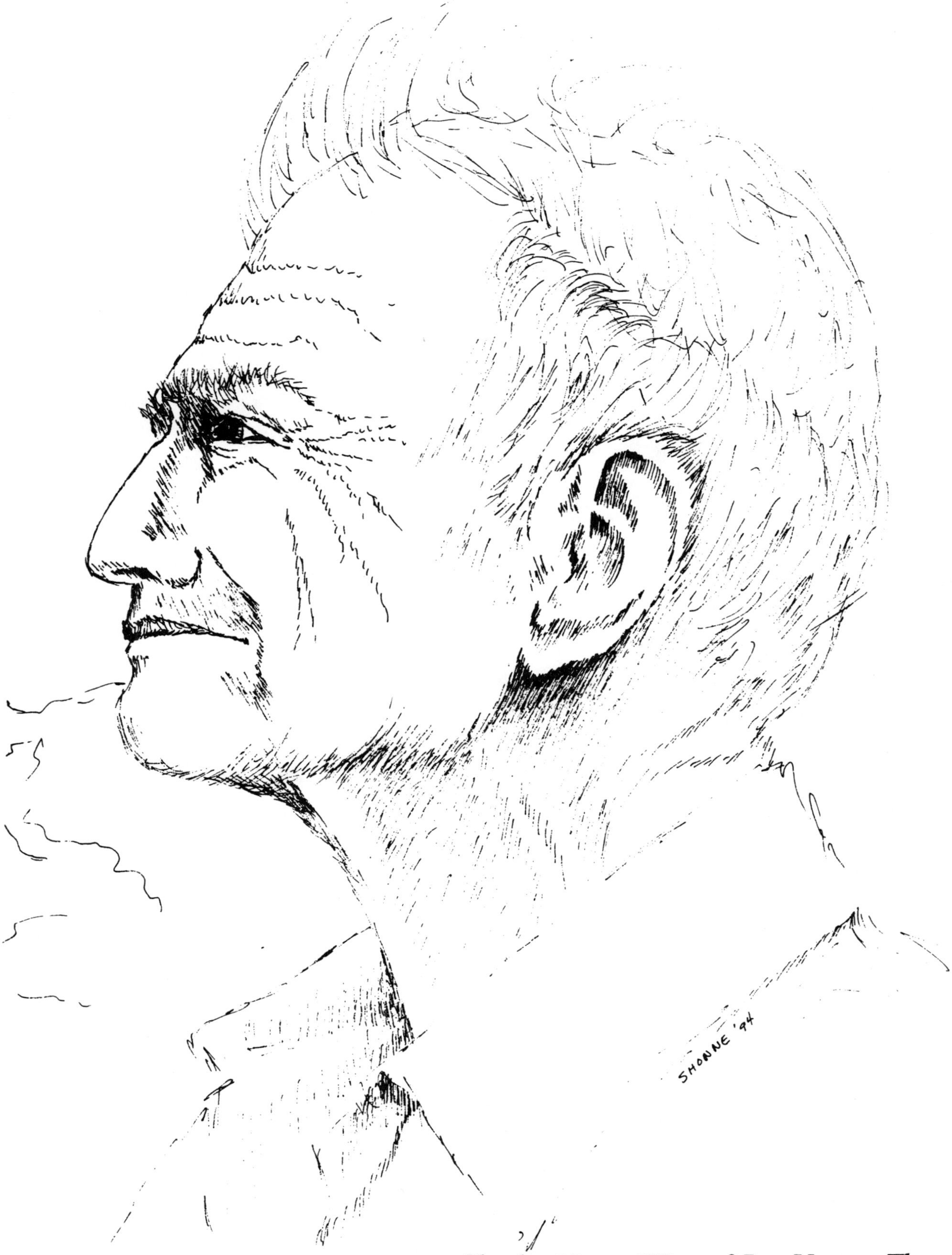

Charles Mraz—"King of Bee Venom Therapy"

❧ PROLOGUE ❧

"A SOUL'S ANSWER TO SUFFERING"

I have been on a journey for many years without realizing it. ❧ As a bird instinctively knows how to fly, I was born with a gift; to give, love and help others. ❧ What I have done all my life has come from deep within me—from my essence, my soul. ❧ I now know that we are all on a journey homeward. ❧ All roads lead home. ❧ This is my story, and since all souls are connected, it is our story. ❧ This book is a mirror. ❧ You will see your reflection in these pages. ❧ Pay special attention to where you see yourself. ❧ You may find that your weaknesses are also your strengths. ❧ This information is important. ❧ It will help you many times. ❧ Remember, we are all suffering: some physically, some emotionally, some spiritually. ❧ We are all trying to find our way home again, back to a time when everything was O.K.

It may appear that this is a book about bees. ❧ It is much more. ❧ This is a book about healing, healing the whole person—body, mind and spirit. ❧ This is a book about healing your life. ❧ We all have a hole within us; an empty place, that yearns to be filled—to be healed. ❧ This book is your companion on your healing journey. ❧ It will help you when you are hurting, confused, discouraged and even when you're hopeful.

I have learned much from the bees. ❧ I am still learning. ❧ I have a burning desire to share this information with you. ❧ This book is a real and concrete way for me to recycle that which I have gained. ❧ The bees flew into my life when I really needed them the most. ❧ I was just coming out of an abusive marriage. ❧ I was feeling alone and discouraged. ❧ Life had very little meaning. ❧ Pat Wagner's story in the Washington Post brought me back to life. ❧ Giving to others was the answer to my prayers. ❧ As I worked with Pat and the bees I received my miracle. ❧ Writing this book is a continuation of my healing process. ❧ The more I give, the more I heal my pain. ❧ I am involving others in my healing process by giving to them. ❧ We all have something to give. ❧ As St. Francis said: "It is in giving, that we receive."

Years ago I had a vision. ❧ I was a Medicine Woman. ❧ I saved my own tears in my "tear-glass bottle" and used those tears to help others in need. ❧ My name became Amber. ❧ Amber was to me the tears of the pine tree. ❧ Under a million years of pressure, they hardened and turned into a precious jewel. ❧ I live my life, turn my suffering into gold, by helping others in need.

Alchemy presents the beautiful image of transforming lead into gold, suffering into beauty. ❧ Alchemists sought "The Pearl of Great Price." ❧ The pearl starts as a grain of sand, an irritant inside the oyster's shell. ❧ The oyster deals with its pain, by covering the grain of sand with a luster, and continuing to do so, day in and day out, until the grain of sand becomes a pearl. ❧ The oyster transforms its suffering into a beautiful jewel.

So it is with our symptoms. ❧ Our pains and our struggles may be the seeds of our greatest treasure. ❧ These seeds may blossom into healing beyond our wildest dreams. ❧ We must befriend our symptoms and our circumstances. ❧ They are not the enemy. ❧ Our problems are a gift from God. ❧ They are here to help us and to teach us. ❧ I never treat symptoms. ❧ I only treat people.

When I was in ninth grade I wrote a career booklet on Physical Therapy. ❧ I called it "Coward Take my Coward's Hand." ❧ I wanted to be a physical therapist because I had been inspired by the book called, "It's Good to be Alive" by Roy Campanella. ❧ Mr. Campanella was the catcher for the Brooklyn Dodgers. ❧ In 1958 a tragic automobile accident left him paralyzed. ❧ He spent the rest of his life in a wheelchair. ❧ I never knew Mr. Campanella personally, but I knew him in my heart. ❧ He was a giant to me. ❧ His story and his positive attitude toward life moved my soul. ❧ He was my hero. ❧ I wanted so desperately to help him. ❧ I have spent my life in my own quiet way trying to help the Roy Campanellas in my life.

As a teenager I was also moved by "The Diary of Anne Frank." ❧ I remember most her belief that people really were "still good at heart" even if they did evil things. ❧ Both Roy Campanella and Anne Frank found a way to rise above their circumstances. ❧ They both found their "Pearl of Great Price."

Is your pain the seed of your pearl? ❧ Is that thorn in your side a friend, not a foe? ❧ Is the illness that's troubling you really a blessing in disguise? ❧ How can you transform the very thing that's at the heart of your suffering into a beautiful jewel? ❧ Only you know the answer to this question. ❧ If your life were a book, what would the title be? ❧ What chapter are you on right now? ❧ Remember, only you can write the next chapter.

What did you come here to do? ❧ What is missing in your life? ❧ Can you do anything about it? ❧ If you could wave a magic wand, how would you use it? ❧ This book is meant to inspire you to greater heights and challenge your greatest fears.

This book is my personal invitation to get to know who you really are, to accept yourself, to fall in love with life again, and to experience the alchemy of turning your suffering into gold.

If I could wave a magic wand right now, I'd wish for you a miracle . . .

Amber Rose

❧ ❧ ❧

THE OLDEST BEE ON THE PLANET WAS FOUND IN FOSSILIZED AMBER, WHICH IS THE SAP OF THE PINE TREE THAT HAS BEEN HARDENED OVER MILLIONS OF YEARS . . .

❧ ❧ ❧

PRAYER ANSWERED

I asked God for strength, that I might achieve,
I was made weak, that I might learn humbly to obey. . .

I asked for health, that I might do greater things,
I was given infirmity, that I might do better things. . .

I asked for riches, that I might be happy,
I was given poverty that I might be wise. . .

I asked for power, that I might have the praise of men,
I was given weakness, that I might feel the need of God. . .

I asked for all things, that I might enjoy life,
I was given life, that I might enjoy all things. . .

I got nothing that I asked for—
But everything that I had hoped for.

Almost despite myself, my unspoiled prayers were
answered.

I am among all men, most richly blessed.

—AUTHOR UNKNOWN, DYING CONFEDERATE SOLDIER

❧ PREFACE ❧

"THE BEST IS YET TO BEE!"

If someone had told me a year and a half ago that I would have a hive in my dining room with 8-10,000 bees, and three beehives in my back yard, I would have told them that they were completely crazy! No way! If that same person had told me that I'd be stinging 20-30 people with honeybees three times a week in my dining room, I would have told them that I'd have to be completely crazy!

Life has the most amazing twists and turns. Just when you think you have it all figured out, something happens to make you question it all over again.

❧ ❧ ❧

"I NOW SEE MY PRACTICE OF APITHERAPY AS A NATURAL AND OBVIOUS EVOLUTION FROM MY TRAINING AS AN ACUPUNCTURIST. I BELIEVE THE BEE STING WAS THE FIRST ACUPUNCTURE NEEDLE."

❧ ❧ ❧

I was an apitherapist waiting to happen. You see, I have been a caretaker all my life. As early as elementary school, I would reach out to the kids with crutches, wheelchairs and hearing aids and invite them to lunch. Well, not too much has really changed since then. Now, instead of inviting them to lunch, I am stinging them with bees at my dining room table. How's that for a quantum leap? Sometimes I even wonder to myself, "How in the world did I get 'here' from 'there'?"

All I know is that I've always loved to help others. I'm always looking for new techniques that work. That's why I became an acupuncturist after being a psychotherapist for many years. Some of my therapy clients were "stuck." They knew why they were upset, but they couldn't break through it. Acupuncture seemed to bring them to a new level of wholeness.

I now see my practice of apitherapy as a natural and obvious evolution from my training as an acupuncturist. However, I believe the bee sting was the first acupuncture needle. Now, as I practice apitherapy, I am simply returning to the original, natural form of acupuncture.

Besides the puncturing of the skin, bee venom therapy and acupuncture have something very special in common. They each strive to stimulate the body's own natural forms of healing. The idea is to get the body to wake up and heal itself. This is not just a band-aid approach to cover up the symptoms or pain of illness. This is a holistic approach: healing the whole person, body, mind and spirit.

So, call it coincidence, or call it fate! Call it being in the right place at the right time. Or call it a miracle waiting to happen. One Tuesday morning in June of 1993, I found myself browsing through the Washington Post. I was looking for a part-time job, while building up my acupuncture practice .

I never made it to the want-ads. This was a very important day for me, one that would change my life forever. Oh, I found a job alright! And it's a full-time job at that. The pay is not very good, but the rewards are great. You see, in the Style section on that Tuesday in June, there was an article called "Hope Stings Eternal." (See Appendix V.) It was an article about Bee Venom Therapy and a remarkable woman named Pat Wagner who has MS.

"IF SOMEONE HAD TOLD ME A YEAR AND A HALF AGO THAT I WOULD HAVE A HIVE IN MY DINING ROOM WITH 8-10,000 BEES, AND THREE BEEHIVES IN MY BACK YARD, I WOULD HAVE TOLD THEM THAT THEY WERE COMPLETELY CRAZY!"

My mission now was crystal clear. I suddenly remembered what I came here to do. A new journey was beginning. I was about to write a new chapter in my life. It seemed as if everything was in slow motion. My whole life made sense.

Sometimes we look for answers in all the wrong places. I was looking for an answer in the want-ad section, but I found so much more in the Style section.

It's scary to think that I could have missed that article completely, or I could have left the paper in the recycling bin where I had tossed it a few hours earlier. But instead, there I was, sitting in my own backyard, unaware that a miracle was about to take place.

"AFTER I READ THE ARTICLE . . . I NOTICED THE BEES AND THE CLOVER ALL AROUND ME. 'MY GOD,' I THOUGHT, 'THE ANSWER TO MY PRAYERS IS HERE IN MY OWN BACKYARD.'"

It was only after I read the article that I noticed the bees and the clover all around me. "My God," I thought, "the answer to my prayers is here in my own backyard." I could actually feel myself taking a new fork in the road. It felt good. I knew my life would never be the same again.

I had heard of Bee Venom Therapy for arthritis many years ago, but the information just went in one ear and out the other. (I guess it was because I didn't know any one suffering with arthritis.) And just several weeks before I read the article in the Post, I had heard about someone using bee stings for MS, and once again I paid no attention.

"BY THE WAY, APITHERAPY IS ALSO MENTIONED IN THE BIBLE, AND IT WAS PRACTICED BY HIPPOCRATES (THE FATHER OF WESTERN MEDICINE). I AM AMAZED THAT EASTERN AND WESTERN CULTURES HAVE INDEPENDENTLY DEVELOPED SIMILAR TECHNIQUES."

But the day after reading the Post article I was at Pat Wagner's doorstep, and I don't even have MS! I watched her placement of stings. "Was she stinging in acupuncture points?" I asked myself. Yes and no. She was stinging mostly on "trigger points," ("hot spots,") and "nerve meridians," (where the nerves come out of the spine and down the arms and legs).

It was obvious to me that any use of acupuncture points was "accidental" or not conscious on her part. She made it clear that she had no formal training in acupuncture and neither did Charles Mraz, the beekeeper who has been doing this for 60 years. Pat was certainly getting very good results. It's funny, I went down to Pat's house thinking there was so much I wanted to teach her, but by the time I left I realized that I had a lot to learn.

Over the next month and a half, I drove down to Southern Maryland three times a week to volunteer with Pat. I saw some pretty amazing and consistent results. And believe me, I knew how incredible this was because I have seen very little success with MS using acupuncture. I began to feel like I was a pioneer in a whole new frontier of medicine.

In late July, Pat was starting to feel burnt out. She decided to take a vacation. All the people who were coming to her house had no idea where they were going to go to get their bee stings. And somehow . . . it just came out of my mouth, "You can come to my house in Bethesda." I MUST HAVE BEEN CRAZY! I didn't even have a beehive! My house was not wheelchair accessible. I didn't even have any special tweezers to catch the bees, which are hard to come by.

I made this commitment on the last Monday in July and I had one week to get it all together. I finally said one day in desperation as I looked up to the heavens, "OK, God . . . You've got to help me do this! I cannot do this by myself." Before I knew it, someone had offered to build the ramp, someone else donated the deposit for the hive, and yet another person gave me eight tweezers.

"CHARLES MRAZ . . . EXPRESSED TO ME (WITH GREAT EXCITEMENT) THAT HE HAD FOUND SEVERAL NEW TRIGGER POINTS ON THE FOOT THAT WERE VERY HELPFUL FOR MS PATIENTS. WITHOUT EXCEPTION, EVERY SINGLE TRIGGER POINT HE SHOWED ME WAS AN ACUPUNCTURE POINT."

That was over a year ago . . . and what a year it has been! Three months after I met Pat Wagner, I was in China attending conferences on apitherapy. The Chinese have been doing "bee-acupuncture" (bee stings in acupuncture points) for over 3000 years to treat a variety of ailments. By the way, apitherapy is also mentioned in the Bible, and it was practiced by Hippocrates (the Father of Western Medicine). I am amazed that Eastern and Western cultures have independently developed similar techniques.

To illustrate the point of how similar these techniques really are, I would like to share the following story: Charles Mraz, considered to be "the King of Bee Venom Therapy" in the United States at this time, expressed to me (with great excitement) that he had found several new trigger points on the foot that were very helpful for MS patients. Without exception, every single trigger point he showed me was an acupuncture point. This confirmed for me the deep similarity and overlap between the two systems of apitherapy. Now, unless you believe in reincarnation and assume that Charles Mraz is a reincarnated acupuncturist from several thousand years ago, the only explanation that I see is that apitherapy is as natural as nature itself. There is a universal truth underlying this system of medicine that must not be ignored. I believe that it is time to elevate apitherapy from just its "folk remedy" status to a viable alternative to the Western medical approach for a wide range of degenerative diseases thought to have an auto-immune or inflammatory basis.

Unfortunately, the kind of therapy described in this book, (BVT and "bee-acupuncture," the use of bee stings in acupuncture points), does not lend itself to the rigorous double-blind controlled studies that are beloved of Western scientists. I'm sure there will be comments that "there is no scientific evidence" for what I am presenting. While doctors are waiting for scientific proof, many patients are getting worse, needlessly. It's sad that the medical community laughs at anecdotal evidence when it arrives from outside Western thinking. True healing is an art which recognizes that each patient is an individual, and rejoices in the glowing faces of those who are better. In true healing, such empirical evidence takes precedence over double-blind procedures which, by their nature, cannot discern the healing in much of alternative or folk medicine.

It is my personal experience that the information in this book is greatly needed. I get hundreds of calls each week seeking information. The main question on everyone's mind is "Where do I sting myself?" By answering that same question day in and day out, I feel as though I am re-inventing the wheel for each person. By writing this book, I am attempting to make this information

"I HAVE SEEN WITH MY OWN EYES WHAT BVT CAN DO. I CONTINUE TO BE INSPIRED AND AMAZED AS MY PATIENTS RECOVER."

more widely accessible and much less costly than trying to get this same information via long distance phone calls to me. The more information the patient has, the more involved he or she can be in the healing process. Knowledge is power. It is very important for the patient to feel as independent as possible. I believe in my heart that this will affect the depth of the healing experience.

I have seen with my own eyes what BVT can do. I continue to be inspired and amazed as my patients recover. I admire their courage and their determination. I am also in awe of these little creatures, the honey bees, that I have come to know and love. I have come to believe that their sweet medicine is truly a gift from God. And although BVT or "bee-acupuncture" has not yet been approved by the F.D.A., there is no question in my mind that it has been approved by the G.O.D.!

"MAY THIS BOOK BE A GENTLE REMINDER TO LIVE EACH DAY AS IF YOUR LIFE DEPENDED ON IT."

It is very important for me to emphasize that this book was not written to convince you to do Bee Venom Therapy. I have written Bee In Balance to share my experience, strength, and hope. May this book be a gentle reminder to live each day as if your life depended on it.

Is there something that someone said to you recently that went in one ear and out the other? Was there something you threw into the recycling bin of your consciousness that you needed to seize and take hold of . . . that might change your life forever . . . ?

If you're not going to do Bee Venom Therapy, what are you going to do with your life? What is that next chapter that you will write for yourself?

May this book encourage you on your journey to wholeness as you take your health back into your own hands.

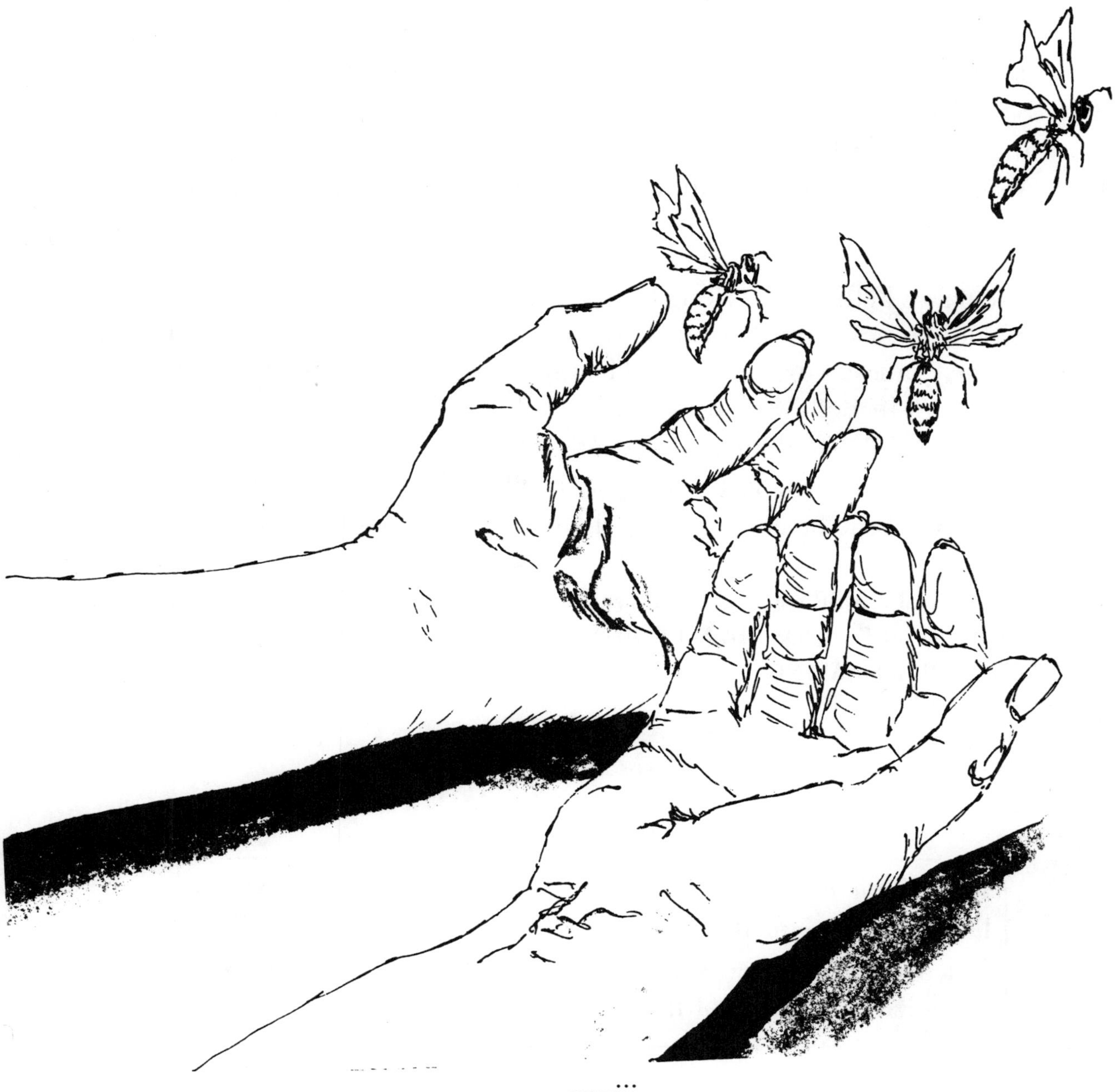

"IT'S NOT ABOUT BEES!"

GEORGE'S STORY

I do not have MS or any other chronic disease. I wanted to get into apitherapy and let the bees get into me. Amber's living room is like a doctor's office, but it isn't. I was impressed by all the people. They came in cars, vans, taxis, scooters, and Red Cross vehicles. Everyone was friendly and talking to one another. There was a lot of love in the room. I was very impressed with one lady who said, "I'm not sick, my body just happens to have MS." I experience community at Amber's home. People are really caring for each other.

It may look like Amber is stinging people with bees. She is doing much more. She gives of herself. How many doctor's do you know that do that? I am loved and cared for by her. This book is about bees, but it's not about bees. What Amber is doing is very simple and yet very profound. I am excited to be part of this process.

The name Bethesda has long been associated with healing. In Biblical times people would come to the Pool of Bethesda to be healed. Bethesda, MD is the home of the National Institutes of Health (NIH). Now, Amber is doing her apitherapy work in Bethesda. It is very special. I believe there is a big difference between what Amber's doing and what's being done at NIH. I believe that Amber is treating the whole person, while NIH is suppressing symptoms with their new drugs. True healing involves the whole person—body, mind, and spirit.

I HAVE BEEN VERY MOVED BY GEORGE'S EXCITEMENT ABOUT THE WORK I AM DOING. HE REMINDS ME SO POIGNANTLY THAT MY WORK IS NOT ABOUT BEES, IT'S ABOUT HEALING. A.R.

> If you have experiences with Bee Venom Therapy you would like to share with the author for use in her next book, "The Jade Bee, and Other Stories," please send them to the address provided at the end of the book.

❧ INTRODUCTION ❧

"HOW WELL ARE YOU WILLING TO BEE?"

PAT WAGNER

The Washington Post newspaper, June 22, 1993 edition, had an exclusive article entitled "Hope Stings Eternal." The story told of things that were happening in Waldorf, Maryland. The paper was tossed aside by Amber Rose without her ever reading about the events described. Later that day, since she was searching for something fulfilling to do with her life at the time, she got the paper out again to look into the classified section. However, she came across "Hope Stings Eternal." She read about honeybee stings being given at my home. She didn't know me but was intrigued by the healing which she was reading about. As an acupuncturist, she wanted to see for herself just what was "buzzing" in the Washington suburb of Waldorf.

Amber came to my house to observe and offer any assistance possible. Well, she wasn't the first nor the last total stranger to appear at my door. However, the others were mostly there to receive bee stings. She was there to learn and help, and that she did. After diligently assisting for weeks on end, she opened her own home to offer bee venom therapy. In her own work, she noticed some relationships to bee sting locations and acupuncture points. To our surprise and excitement, we discovered that acupuncture can, even after many hours, reactivate the body's reaction to distant bee stings related via the acupuncture meridians!

With that excitement, we considered jointly writing a book to inform people of the many miracles out there just waiting to be discovered. Since I am not familiar with any detailed aspects of acupuncture, we decided to write separate books yet explain the joint usefulness of these two means of healing oneself. She has kindly asked me to submit for inclusion in her book my bee sting suggestions regarding the apitherapy part of healing. The two can work nicely together.

My upcoming guide, "How Well Are You Willing To Bee?," will hopefully give you some pointers, some knowledge, and some interesting reading as you strive for improved health. Through this book by my friend, Amber Rose, it is my hope that you will . . .

DISCOVER A MIRACLE!

Apitheraply yours,

Pat Wagner
"The Bee Lady"

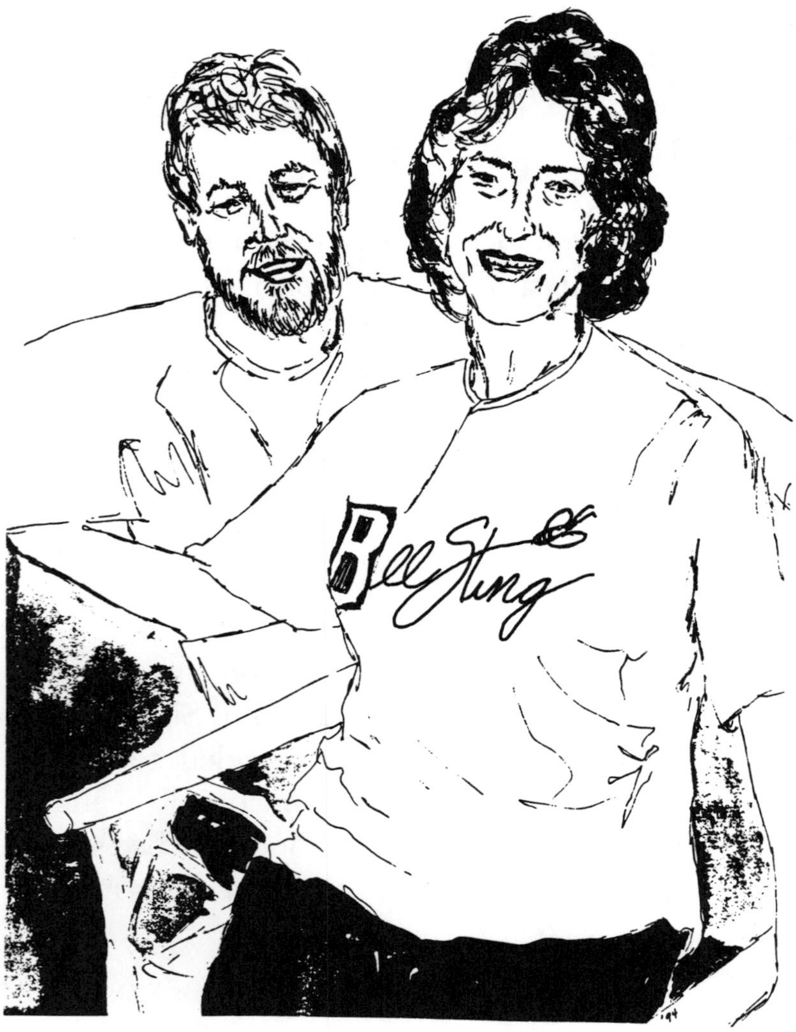

This is Pat Wagner—"The Bee Lady" and her husband "Sting Ray."

DISCLAIMER

This book is for educational purposes only. It is not intended to present or prescribe any therapy or treatment for any person. Nor is it intended to be used for the diagnosis of any disease or condition, whether that diagnosis be consistent with Western or Eastern thought.

I cannot make any medical claims for BVT. All I can share is my story and the stories of those courageous people who have decided to take control of their lives in a new way.

Those who seek to put the information in this book into practice do so based upon their own knowledge and skills and must take full responsibility for their efforts. The author does not assume any responsibility for injury or harm resulting from the use or misuse of this information. The author is available for consultation to ensure the proper use of this information. See information form on page 214.

Patients with medical symptoms or who believe they have a health care condition should consult a physician to obtain a diagnosis and to consider any options that Western medicine has for their condition. Patients may also wish to consult with their physician before undertaking any of the approaches outlined in this book.

BEFORE ATTEMPTING ANY STINGS FOR YOURSELF OR ANYONE ELSE, MAKE SURE THAT YOU OBTAIN A BEE STING KIT AND KNOW HOW TO USE IT.

It is important to understand that Oriental medicine, of which Acupuncture is one branch, approaches health and illness from a different paradigm than Western medicine. Oriental diagnosis does not conform to Western diagnostic categories, and those with the same Western diagnosis, such as MS, may have very different Oriental diagnoses, and thus different "bee-acupuncture" treatment plans.

Making a complete and accurate Oriental diagnosis requires extensive training and personal contact with the patient. This book is not intended to supplant that process, but to provide information so that those using honeybees may do so skillfully and add to the impact of their work.

It is VERY IMPORTANT that you read and follow the information provided in the section called "Reactions," found on page xxxix, and the section called "Warnings," page xlii, before you attempt to follow any practice outlined in this book.

CONVENTIONS:

(caduceus)	The CADUCEUS symbol is placed near warnings or other medical information. It is important that you read and pay special attention to this material.
source point[G]	This book provides a GLOSSARY in Appendix I. Some of the terms used in this book, such as source point, come from acupuncture theory. Words marked with a[G] are defined in the glossary.
F	Points which are FORBIDDEN to sting are marked with an F. You will note this symbol on the lists of points found in Chapter 7. These points can be used for acupressure.
Gender	While an effort has been made to remain gender-neutral, references are occasionally made to either "he" or "she." The references are made in an effort to balance considerations of grammar with that of equity.

REACTIONS

One amazing reaction to bee stings is that you might get well. You should also know, however, that there are four kinds of reactions to bee stings:

1. Generalized Immediate✚
2. Localized Immediate
3. Generalized Delayed
4. Localized Delayed

A definition of the word generalized is: a systemic reaction, meaning you get stung in one place and you have a reaction somewhere else.

A definition of localized is: you get a reaction in or near the site where you were stung.

GENERALIZED IMMEDIATE✚

This is the only reaction to bee stings that is LIFE-THREATENING. Within the first 1-5 minutes the person has a generalized reaction to the stings. They may have a feeling of malaise, severe itching all over the body (even the palms and the scalp), or develop a reddening of the skin. (I use liquid Benadryl in this situation.) Up until this point, the reaction is not life threatening. If however, this reaction continues on to DIFFICULTY BREATHING and HEART FAILURE, this is called "ANAPHYLACTIC SHOCK." This process generally occurs within 6 to 10 minutes. If the person develops difficulty breathing, use your "BEE STING KIT" IMMEDIATELY. This kit is an epinephrine auto-injector that is prescribed for you by a physician. It is wise to read the instructions and know how to use the kit before you begin with your test sting.

LOCALIZED IMMEDIATE

This is not a life-threatening reaction. The person feels the immediate sensation of the bee sting in the area where he or she was stung. It feels like a spicy burn for approximately 1-2 minutes. The pain of the sting can be reduced by applying ice (or a frozen metal can) to the area prior to and after the stinging, and massaging the area immediately after the person has been stung.

GENERALIZED DELAYED

There is no risk to life with a generalized delayed reaction. This is a systemic reaction that affects the overall body (malaise, nausea, light-headedness, stiffness, itching or hives) and occurs more than an hour after the treatment. This is the time to listen to your body; if you feel like resting, then rest. Don't push yourself. A "Healing Crisis," see definition below and in Chapter 1, may be a form of generalized delayed reaction.

LOCALIZED DELAYED

You can have a delayed reaction to the bee sting that is in the area surrounding the site of the sting. An example of a localized delayed reaction would be redness, swelling, itching, heat, or blisters close to where you were stung. This is uncomfortable, but certainly not life-threatening. This is actually a very positive sign that the body's immune system is waking up.

WHAT IS A GOOD REACTION?

The following reactions are positive signs that your immune system is waking up:

- REDNESS, SWELLING, AND A LOT OF ITCHING IN THE AREAS WHERE YOU WERE STUNG. THIS IS THE LOCAL ALLERGIC REACTION THAT IS NOT LIFE THREATENING. Although you may not enjoy this, it is a positive sign. It means that your immune system is awake. If you do not get this reaction it means that your immune system is very suppressed. A seasoned apitherapist is very encouraged when he or she sees a big red reaction. ("The bigger the better!") It is possible that this reaction may continue for a month or so. Preparation H, or some equivalent, seems to work well for itching. If you take something orally for the itching, it may counteract the effects of the venom. That is why we generally recommend something topical.

- "HEALING CRISIS." Somewhere between the first and the fifth bee sting treatment you may notice some flu-like symptoms: fatigue, nausea, stiffness, tired and achy muscles, perhaps even a high fever. You may not want to get out of bed or go through your usual daily routine. Don't despair. This will usually last

3-4 days at most. As is often the case with any trauma, the day after the stings may be the worst. Remember, it is a good sign that toxins are leaving your system and being flushed out through the bloodstream. So, the healing crisis will not last forever. You have to push through it. You may cut down on your number of stings for a treatment or two, and then build back up again. Remember this is normal and is nothing to worry about. When you are not feeling well you may be tempted to give up, but I urge you to continue. Remember "this too shall pass."

➻ ENERGY. One of the first things that many people report with the bee stings is increased energy. Enjoy it! Your body, mind and spirit have been asleep. This is a real wake-up call. The adrenal glands are stimulated by the venom and this may result in an adrenaline rush. The body is working better because you have more energy and this may lift your spirits.

➻ FEELING THE STINGS. Let's look at the positive side; if the bee stings may hurt for the first minute or two, at least you can feel them. If at first you are numb and you don't feel the stings, that means your nerve endings are "asleep." So, even though it is painful to feel the stings, the good news is that you are feeling something. This means your body is waking up.

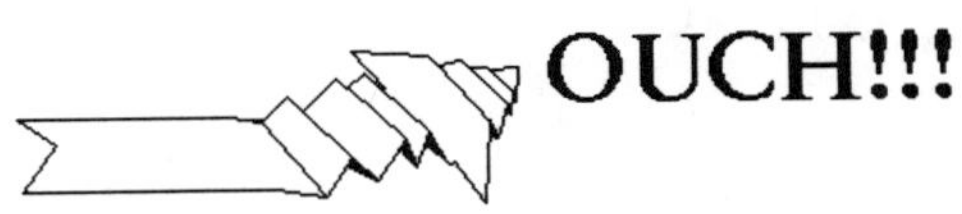

➻ FEELING EXCITED ABOUT DOING THE BEE STINGS AND ABOUT LIFE IN GENERAL. Some people notice a natural high and a sense of well being. This is a very positive sign. You have started on a new adventure.

THE HONEYBEE MAY VISIT AS MANY AS 100 FLOWERS AS IT COLLECTS NECTAR AND POLLEN DURING A TRIP AWAY FROM THE HIVE . . .

WARNINGS

"BEE—SMART"

✓ You may get well!

✓ You may walk better!

✓ You may have better bladder control!

✓ You may be able to sleep through the night!

✓ You may have more energy!

✓ You may have better balance!

"SAFE—STINGING"

✓ Before doing anything, obtain a bee sting kit and learn how to use it.

✓ Some people really are allergic to honeybees, but this is exceedingly rare. Most people mistakenly believe they are allergic for the following reasons:

- When they get stung on the hand, their arm swells up, gets red and itches a lot.

- They stepped on a nest of bees as a child or when they were mowing the lawn and had a strong reaction.

- They were told that they were allergic to bees.

In reality, when you get stung on the hand and your arm swells up, and gets red and itchy, this is a good sign. It means that your immune system is working. If you had a bad reaction after "stepping on a nest of bees" you were probably stung by yellow jackets and not honeybees, because honeybees do not live in the ground. If you were told that you are allergic to all bees because you are allergic to yellow jackets and/or a wasps, this is not accurate; it does not mean that you are allergic to honeybees.

✓ The only way you really know for sure if you are allergic to honeybees is to get a test sting. IF YOU HAVE TROUBLE BREATHING WITHIN THE FIRST 5-10 MINUTES AFTER BEING STUNG, THEN YOU ARE ALLERGIC TO HONEYBEES. YOU WILL NEED TO USE THE BEE STING KIT (epinephrine and anti-histamine) PRESCRIBED BY YOUR DOCTOR. BE SURE YOU READ THE DIRECTIONS ON THE PACKAGE BEFORE YOU GET YOUR TEST STING. (See "Reactions.") REMEMBER, THE ONLY REACTION TO BEE STINGS THAT IS LIFE THREATENING IS A GENERALIZED IMMEDIATE REACTION THAT QUICKLY DEVELOPS INTO BREATHING PROBLEMS.

✓ Bee stings hurt. You may want to use ice to numb the area you are about to sting. This reduces the pain. Bee stings do feel like a spicy burn for a minute or so. You can also place ice near the area while the stinger is in, but it is best not to put the ice right on top of the stinger.

✓ Start with one test sting and take it out immediately. This is often done on the knee because it is far away from the heart, but not too low on the extremities (which tend to swell a lot if you do them too early). If you feel OK after 10-15 minutes proceed with two to five more stings. Remover the stingers 10-15 minutes later taking care to pull the stingers out sideways along the skin, not straight upward. I recommend that you stay away from the extremities (the arms and legs) at first, because they tend to swell more than the rest of the body, especially at the beginning.

✓ It is important to increase slowly the number of stings you get. I usually start with 3-6 stings the first time, depending on the severity of the condition. With a chronic illness I usually start by giving six stings the first two sessions, then I increase the number of stings by two every other session. It is very important not to jump from eight stings to fourteen stings. Don't give the body more than it can handle too quickly or too early. Remember "slow and steady wins the race." You'll probably be doing bee stings for quite a while, so "take it easy." I have found 15-20 stings per session is a good maximum. If you have a chronic condition I recommend that you commit to stinging yourself 3 times a week for 6 months.

✓ It is important not to give up too soon. You may be tempted to stop the bee stings if you don't notice changes right away. Please don't lose sight of the fact that you have a chronic illness. You didn't get this way overnight and there is no magic pill that will cure you overnight. Healing is a process that takes time.

✓ IF YOU HAVE STOPPED THE BEE STINGS FOR MORE THAN TWO WEEKS FOR ANY REASON, ALWAYS START WITH ONE TEST STING. AFTER 15 MINUTES YOU CAN PROCEED, BUT DO NOT START AT THE LEVEL WHERE YOU LEFT OFF. START WITH JUST A FEW STINGS AND WORK YOUR WAY BACK UP.

✓ I am aware of one case where a man who had been drinking heavily went into anaphylactic shock upon receiving bee stings. Therefore, I RECOMMEND NOT CONSUMING ALCOHOLIC BEVERAGES OR RECREATIONAL DRUGS WHILE DOING BEE VENOM THERAPY.

✓ There are conflicting reports about BVT and PREGNANCY. Some people say it helps fertility and others say it may cause miscarriages. I recommend avoiding bee venom therapy while pregnant.

✓ DO NOT DO BVT WITHOUT ADEQUATE VITAMIN C. It is highly recommended that you take 2-3000 milligrams of Vitamin C daily. Bee stings stimulate the adrenal glands to make cortisol, but the adrenal glands need Vitamin C to do this. (The importance of cortisol is discussed in Chapter 1.)

✓ If you are stinging someone else, you may want to consider using a written consent form. (See Appendix IV for a sample.)

HOW TO USE THIS BOOK

✓ This is a comprehensive textbook. It may be read on different levels. This book will help both the beginner who is just getting started with bee venom therapy (BVT), as well as the person who has been doing BVT for a while. It is written for the person who is being stung and the person doing the stinging. It is for both the lay person and the health practitioner who may want to incorporate some of this work into their practice. This book can also be read by anyone who just wants to learn more about the philosophy of the five elements of oriental medicine.

The following information will help you decide which chapters will be the most important ones for you:

✓ If you are a beginner, you'll be reading this book to learn more about BVT and where to sting yourself or others. I recommend you start with Part 1. If you are interested in trying "bee-acupuncture," go on to Part 2. If not, skip Part 2 for now and go on to Part 3, which suggests other modalities to combine with your BVT work. Read the directions below that highlight the parts of the book you want to read.

✓ If you have been doing BVT for a while and you are looking for new places to sting yourself or others, you may want to try "bee-acupuncture," the use of bee stings in acupuncture points. If this is the case, I recommend you read the entire book.

✓ If your sole purpose for reading this book is to have a better understanding of Chinese medicine and the five elements of nature, and you are not planning to sting yourself or others, you may want to start with Chapter 4 and then go on to Part 2. If you are a health practitioner this information may give you new ideas for creating treatment plans for acupuncture, acupressure, massage therapy, psychotherapy or other healing arts. If this information intrigues you, I encourage you to read the rest of the book. Even if you are not planning to do BVT or "bee-acupuncture" yourself, you may know someone who could benefit from this amazing and wonderful treatment.

DIRECTIONS

INTRODUCTORY MATERIALS

IT IS VERY IMPORTANT THAT YOU READ THE SECTION CALLED REACTIONS. This will explain the four different kinds of reactions that may result from Bee Venom Therapy (Generalized Immediate, Localized Immediate, Generalized Delayed, and Localized Delayed). It explains that the Generalized Immediate is the only reaction that could be life threatening. It also describes what a good reaction to BVT might look like. This section of the book is of utmost importance. It is followed by a section entitled "Warnings," which describes the necessity for a bee sting kit for all persons doing BVT and when to use it. It describes how to give a test sting, remove the stinger, and how to choose how many stings to do and how quickly to increase the number of stings.

PART 1—HONEYBEES

CHAPTER 1 gives you a basic understanding of the common questions and answers about BVT.

In CHAPTER 2 gives you instructions that will help you get started. It will teach you how to get bees, how to keep them alive, how to give yourself a test sting, and how and when to remove the stinger. Also discussed is what you might experience during your healing process and how medications may affect BVT.

CHAPTER 3 explains the five basic places to sting yourself: "trigger points," "nerve meridians," acupuncture pathways, acupuncture points, and scars. Do this for the first month. (If you have a serious/chronic illness, it is recommended that you continue stinging yourself for a minimum of six months, three times per week.)

CHAPTER 4, WE ARE ALL DOROTHYS AND TOTOS, AND WE ARE JUST TRYING TO FIND OUR WAY HOME, explains that all sickness is homesickness and that we are all trying to find our way back to a time when we felt healthy and centered. This chapter presents a whole new way of looking at your "illness," and beyond your "illness." It encourages you to let this book be your guide on your journey back toward health.

PART 2—ORIENTAL MEDICINE

After you have experienced stinging yourself on "trigger points" and "nerve meridians," you may want to explore acupuncture pathways and acupuncture points. The following chapters will help you decide which pathways and points to use.

CHAPTER 5 describes the basic philosophy of acupuncture and introduces the concept of the five elements. Understanding the interaction of the five elements in creating harmony or disharmony helps one choose the proper "bee-acupuncture" treatment.

CHAPTER 6 begins the heart of the oriental approach to healing. This practical chapter is where you will learn about the Five Elements of Nature: WOOD, FIRE, EARTH, METAL, AND WATER. These elements are the foundation of Chinese Medicine. The goal of this chapter is to first help you select which one of the five elements needs the most attention. This will be the element where you will begin your work. The selection process continues as you select which pathway you want to work on first. Each element has two pathways that go with it, except for the fire element which has four. This second step will help you pick which pathway is most out of balance on the element you have chosen.

CHAPTER 7 will provide you with specific treatment plans, illustrations and point names for each of the pathways. You can apply these treatment plans to the pathway(s) which need attention.

CHAPTER 8 describes two extra pathways that are not ruled by the five elements: the conception vessel and the governor vessel. It shows you when to use these pathways and gives you a treatment plan for each. This chapter also describes special points which you might find useful.

CHAPTER 9 you will find discussion of six major blocks that might be preventing you from getting the best results with BVT. An explanation is given about how these blocks might be corrected by bee stings and/or acupuncture.

PART 3—COMMON SENSE

CHAPTER 10 will help you if you've been receiving the bee stings for a while and feel like you aren't getting better. It gives many suggestions you can either put into action or at least think about. This is a good chapter to look at or review if you are feeling discouraged or confused.

CHAPTER 11 is written for you if you are stinging someone else. It explains what you can expect. This chapter has helpful suggestions on how to involve the patient in the total healing process and how to sting with your heart, not just your mind. This supportive chapter will help if you are feeling confused or discouraged.

CHAPTER 12 will give you ideas of how you can improve your results with BVT or "bee-acupuncture" through nutrition and an exploration of food allergies. It includes what kinds of foods are healthy for you, what herbs and supplements you may want to explore, and what kinds of foods you might want to stay away from.

CHAPTER 13 will give you other suggestions that may increase the effectiveness of the bee stings. It briefly describes topics such as meditation, exercise, massage, Bach Flower remedies, and keeping a positive attitude.

APPENDIX

Appendix I: A GLOSSARY follows the conclusion with simple definitions of terms that are used over and over again in the book. Terms in the glossary which are used without an explanation are marked[G] to let you know that an explanation can be found in the glossary.

Appendix II: After the glossary you will find a recommended READING LIST and a list of videotapes that are available. This is followed by USEFUL NAMES AND ADDRESSES of helpful organizations and people.

Appendix III provides more technical detail on a variety of subjects, such as the specific technical details of what is in bee venom, what illnesses seem to respond well to BVT anecdotally, and more information the other products found in the hive.

Appendix IV includes forms you may need.

Appendix V is a reprint of an article originally published in the Washington Post on June 22, 1993, called "Hope Stings Eternal," reprinted with permission.

This book is not meant to be a definitive answer to how this therapy "should" be done. What is presented here is just one way of approaching the subject matter. My intention is to create a comprehensive text that will help the beginner get started, stimulate the creativity of point selection for those who have been doing this for a while, and to challenge the health care practitioner to look at the world and their patients in a whole new way. I am also attempting to give the reader an overview of the Five Elements of Chinese medicine and to bridge the gap between the Eastern and Western approach to using honeybees for healing. I hope you find it helpful.

PART 1

HONEYBEES

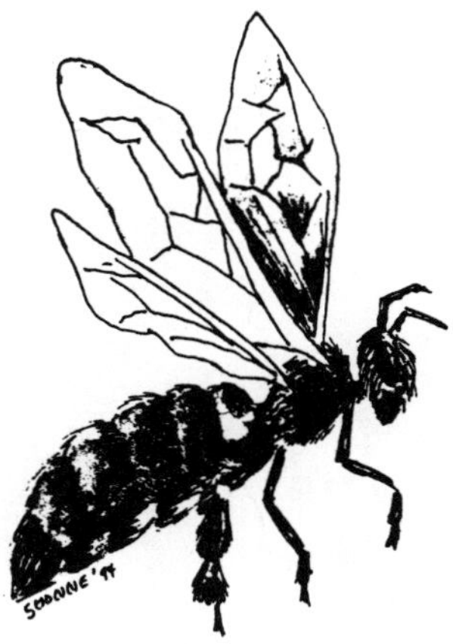

CHAPTER 1

COMMON QUESTIONS AND ANSWERS

Every day I get calls from people full of questions about bees and bee venom therapy. The most common question is "Where do I sting myself?" The book you are holding in your hands is my effort to answer that question in a way I hope will hold your attention and help you learn how to take care of your own health. The answers to the following commonly asked questions will help us get started:

WHAT IS "BEE VENOM THERAPY (BVT)?"

BVT is the use of live bee stings (or injectable venom) to treat various diseases such as arthritis, multiple sclerosis (MS), lupus, sciatica, low back pain, and tennis elbow to name just a few. (A more complete list of "anecdotal reports" can be found in the Appendix III.) BVT refers to any use of bee venom to assist the body in healing itself.

WHAT IS "BEE—ACUPUNCTURE?"

"Bee-acupuncture" is the use of live bee stings in acupuncture points for treating a variety of illnesses. This therapy has been practiced in China for 3-5000 years. "Bee-acupuncture" is thus a specific type of BVT or apitherapy. In this book, "bee-acupuncture" is occasionally used interchangeably with BVT and apitherapy.

WHAT IS "APITHERAPY?"

Apitherapy ("Apis" is Latin for "bee") is the use of honeybee products for medicinal purposes. This would include: bee venom, raw honey, royal jelly, pollen, propolis, and beeswax.

WHAT ARE THE HEALTH BENEFITS OF USING THE BEE PRODUCTS FROM THE HIVE, OTHER THAN BEE VENOM?

RAW HONEY is powerful medicine both externally and internally. Externally it is good for sterile, painless wound and burn dressings, as well as bedsores. Raw honey draws water from the environment and kills germs. It contains an anti-bacterial enzyme called glucose oxidase, which converts to hydrogen peroxide. Internally, raw honey is a good substitute for sugar; it gives you natural energy and it helps with constipation, insomnia and obesity. Drops of raw honey in the eyes have been used to treat cataracts.

❧ ❧ ❧

THE ROMAN GOD OF LOVE AND ROMANCE (CUPID) DIPPED HIS ARROWS IN HONEY. . .

❧ ❧ ❧

BEE POLLEN is derived from the most vital part of the plant and brought back to the hive by the bees. It is the primary protein source for the "busy bees." It is considered by many to be the world's most perfect food. It is chock full of amino acids (which proteins are made of), vitamins, and minerals. Pollen has been known to be helpful for allergies, low blood pressure, goiter, respiratory problems, issues with the immune system, and mental strain. It is thought to have antibiotic qualities as well.

❧ ❧ ❧

BEES COMMUNICATE WITH OTHER BEES WITH THEIR PHEROMONES (SCENTS) AND THROUGH DANCE . . . THE DANCING MOVEMENTS LET OTHER BEES KNOW THE LOCATION OF THE POLLEN AND THE NECTAR . . .

❧ ❧ ❧

ROYAL JELLY is what the nurse bees feed to the larva that have been selected to become queen bees. Royal jelly has a supply of gamma globulin, which helps fight infections and stimulate the immune system. It also contains decanoic acid that helps stimulate antibiotic activity in the body. Royal jelly has been known to be helpful for varicose veins, stress and mental exhaustion, sexual deficiencies, infertility, depression, anxiety, gastroduodenal ulcers, skin problems, Parkinson's Disease, high triglyceride levels, and blood pressure, as well as arresting tumor growth.

PROPOLIS is also known as "Russian Penicillin." Propolis is a natural antibiotic. Bee propolis is a resinous substance that the bees gather from the bark and leaf buds of trees. Propolis has been around for 45 million years. It is used by the bees to glue down loose parts of the hive. Propolis makes the hive sterile. Propolis is often used with success for sore throats, allergies, periodontal problems, ulcers, burns, bruises, nasal and respiratory problems.

BEESWAX has been used for centuries for candles, but it is also helpful for burns. It is one of the ingredients in a new moist exposed burn ointment (MEBO) being used successfully in China for treatment of severe burns and surface ulcers. MEBO cuts the healing time and shortens the hospital stay of burn victims by one third. Patients are pain-free within minutes of the application. MEBO also eliminates infections. 72% of all burn victims who die in the United States, die of infections.

According to Professor Harry Gaynor, President of the National Burn Victim Foundation, MEBO has been tested in an F.D.A. certified laboratory for safety and toxicity. It has passed the tests with flying colors. It has also been used successfully on over 600,000 patients in China. Based on these results, 8 hospitals are ready to go to clinical trials. However, they are prevented by F.D.A. standards which require prior testing on burnt four-legged rats to establish efficacy of the product. According to Gaynor,"600,000 human beings should far outweigh 200 furry rats to be burned in order to prove the value of the product." However, the F.D.A. does have its standards. Pakistan, Germany, France, and Israel are very interested and plan to send doctors to China to learn to use MEBO.

WHAT IS THE HISTORY OF APITHERAPY?

Apitherapy can be traced back to ancient China in the East and to Hippocrates in the West. It is even mentioned in the Bible and the Koran. Apitherapy or BVT is being practiced all over the world. The history of apitherapy/BVT in the U.S. goes back almost 100 years. It was practiced by several prominent doctors including Dr. Bodog Beck, who started treating people in his New York City office in the late 1920's. Dr. Beck's book, "Bee Venom Therapy," has been a classic for 60 years. Two of Dr. Beck's students were Dr. Raymond L. Carey from Hollywood, California, and Dr. P.H. O'Connell of Norwich, Connecticut. Dr. Beck died in 1942 and Dr. Carey and Dr. O'Connell carried on their work for approximately 50 years.

The last surviving student of Dr. Beck is a Middlebury, Vermont beekeeper named Charles Mraz, who is almost 90 years old. He has been practicing apitherapy/BVT for over 60 years, with remarkable results. He is known by many as the "King of BVT" and I even heard a woman from Michigan say, "Where I come from, you are known as 'God'." Without a doubt, Charles Mraz has kept BVT and apitherapy alive in the US. Most of his experience has been with treating arthritis, but his recent success with MS victims has catapulted apitherapy into the limelight. The success of this therapy for many patients has been documented on many of the major television networks and major newspapers in the U.S. in the last year.

WHAT IS IN BEE VENOM?

Bee venom is made up of at least 18 pharmacologically active components. Three of the main ingredients are: Melittin (which has powerful antibacterial and anti-inflammatory properties), Adolapin (which has analgesic, as well as anti-inflammatory properties), and Apamin (which produces an anti-inflammatory response without compromising the body's immune system). Apamin may be the primary active ingredient in the treatment of multiple sclerosis. In the case of MS, many symptoms result from inflammatory degeneration of the nerve sheaths that carry electrical signals to and from the brain. Nerve impulses become blocked when the sheath degenerates, because it doesn't conduct electricity very well. Apamin doesn't stop the degeneration, but it seems to improve the conductivity of the degenerating sheath. It seems that Apamin is what MS patients need to get nerve impulses down to the muscles. Bee venom contains a remarkable number of active ingredients. These compounds are detailed in Appendix III.

HOW DOES BEE VENOM THERAPY WORK?

When you get stung by a honeybee, your body has to deal with the foreign substance that has entered it. Bee venom doesn't cure anything, but it stimulates the body to heal itself. Although scientists are not really sure exactly how BVT works, it is believed that the bee venom stimulates the adrenal glands to "wake up" and produce cortisol. Cortisol is the body's own natural form of cortisone, and is produced as part of a complex cascade of reactions the body orchestrates in its own wisdom. The most positive healing comes from this complete and natural response, rather than by injecting the body with an isolated and synthetic form of cortisone.

In addition, bee stings create a fever (redness and heat) in the area where you were stung. This fever breaks down the bee venom. Hippocrates (the father of medicine in the West) said, "Give me a fever and I can cure all illness." One way that the body breaks down the bee venom (which is a foreign protein) is by heating up the area.

The body also dilutes the venom by bringing fluid to the area (swelling). The blood washes away the by-products of this process. When new blood returns to the area the patient often experiences itching. The swelling, heat, and itching are all positive signs that the BVT is working. This process helps cleans up the underlying problem as well as the venom, "killing two birds with one bee."

The underlying problem or chronic condition is healed by the body's reaction to the bee sting (an acute condition). This is consistent with the teachings of Hahneman (the Father of Homeopathy), who said: "You can never cure a chronic condition; you must make it acute."

Somewhere between the first and the fifth treatment the patient may develop flu-like symptoms: fatigue, fever, headache, body aches, nausea, and even diarrhea. This is a "healing crisis" and is a good sign. The only way out of this is through it! Usually, a "healing crisis" lasts a few days, but it varies from person to person and may linger for several weeks. Imagine that your car is stuck in a snow drift. You try and try to get it out by going back and forth . . . back and forth . . . . Eventually, you get enough momentum and your car goes over the edge of the snow drift and you are "home free!" This is the way it is sometimes with the "healing crisis." You take a few bee stings, and then a few more, and then finally you have a real "healing crisis." When this happens, keep rocking the car! It is important not to give up at this time, because you may be about to break free. If you feel the need, you can slightly reduce the number of stings during this time.

Some people feel tempted to give up during the "healing crisis." Try to continue. Some people stop and then come back a week and a half later to try again. After one test sting, I give them a few more and see how they do. To their amazement, the reaction is often very mild and they do not get the flu-like symptoms as before. As previously noted in the warnings section, if you are away from the bee stings for more than two weeks, you should always start with one test sting and proceed slowly.

IF I AM ALLERGIC TO BEES, CAN I DO BEE VENOM THERAPY?

Most people who say they are allergic to bees usually mean that they swell, get red and itch in the area where they were stung. As described earlier, this is a good reaction to bee venom. This happens because the body's immune system is breaking down the foreign substance. (See "Reactions.") Remember, the only life-threatening reaction to bee venom is anaphylactic shock. (See "Warnings.")

If you "stepped on a hive" when you were a kid and got stung many times you were probably stung by yellow jackets. If you go into anaphylactic shock with yellow jackets or wasps this does not mean that the same thing will happen with honeybees. The only way to know for sure is to try one test sting. If it turns out that you do go into anaphylactic shock from honeybee venom, and you want to do BVT, I recommend that you find an experienced person who can desensitize you. This is done with very small amounts of venom over a period of time. Do not attempt to do this yourself.

CAN I BECOME ALLERGIC TO HONEYBEES WHILE DOING BVT?

It is highly unlikely that you will become allergic to honeybees during a course of BVT. Actually, the opposite is true. The more stings you get overtime, the less likely you are to develop an anaphylactic shock reaction. The more stings you get, the less redness, swelling, and itching too. If you come off some of your medication, you may need to adjust your number of stings. 20 bee stings when you're on your medicine may feel OK, but the same 20 stings when you come off your medicine may feel like too much. You may decide to drop the number of stings down for a while as you cut down on your medication.

WHAT DO I NEED TO DO WHILE I AM DOING BEE VENOM THERAPY?

It is strongly recommended that you take 2-3000 milligrams of Vitamin C daily while you are doing BVT. This is a much larger dose of Vitamin C than you will get from drinking orange juice. For example, an 8 ounce glass of fresh squeezed orange juice has 129 milligrams of Vitamin C. One orange has 75 milligrams. Vitamin C comes in many forms: capsules, chewable tablets and liquid. You can also get a buffered form if you find that it upsets your stomach. If you take mega-doses of Vitamin C, it is a good idea to spread the dose out over the day; it's also important to taper off rather than suddenly quit. It is also wise to eat whole, natural foods rather than white sugar, white flour products, dairy products, and saturated fats. Some people may be allergic to these or other foods; these allergies can add to the difficulty in allowing a natural healing regimen like bee stings to be effective. To allow your body a chance to heal, I also recommend that you abstain from alcoholic beverages and cigarettes. Some other nutritional supplements that might be beneficial include: honey bee products (raw, unheated, unfiltered honey; royal jelly; pollen; and propolis), a good Vitamin B complex, Vitamin B-12 shots, Vitamin E, magnesium, zinc and other minerals. Be sure that you are getting enough protein.

You may also want to consider prayer, meditation, yoga, and some kind of exercise. Massage therapy and/or acupuncture treatments might also prove beneficial.

IS IT OK TO TREAT YOURSELF EVERYDAY?

Although there is no rule cast in stone, I highly recommend that you don't sting yourself everyday. It is important to give the body a rest from the stings and a chance to heal. There is also another theory that if you sting yourself everyday, then your body gets lazy and doesn't learn to do things for itself; it relies on the bee venom too much.

WHAT IS THE PROPER LENGTH OF TREATMENT FOR BEE VENOM THERAPY?

If you have a serious or chronic illness, it is recommended that you do the bee stings for at least six months, three times per week. Remember, your body is healing itself during the interval between stings. If your body is really depleted it may take a long time to rebuild your energy. You didn't get this way overnight, and you are not going to be healed overnight. Nature heals slowly. Nature takes her time, while teaching us patience.

If you are treating a problem that is more recent and less severe, like a pulled muscle or a stiff neck, then a shorter course of treatment is more appropriate.

DOES IT REALLY MATTER WHERE YOU ARE STUNG?

It is not known whether the actual site of the bee sting is important. Charles Mraz has been stinging people on "trigger points/hot spots" and "nerve meridians" for 60 years with very good results. The Chinese have been stinging people on acupuncture points for over 3000 years with great success. Other's say the site of the sting doesn't matter because the bee venom's effects are systemic. Therefore, all you need to do is get the venom into the system over a period of time. I believe that bee venom has strong systemic effects, but that its power is heightened by locating the stings in specific points.

IS BEE VENOM A TREATMENT OR A CURE?

The answer to this is unknown. There are many reports that patients with arthritis, shingles, scleroderma, and other ailments have experienced "cures." On the other hand, it appears that BVT is more of a "treatment" for MS than a "cure." It seems that the venom stimulates the adrenal glands for a few days, after which symptoms may return if BVT is not continued. An example of this would be a patient who is doing well and then is unable to do her bee stings for a week because her beekeeper is out of town. By the end of the week the patient is feeling stiff and having trouble walking. Then her beekeeper returns and she gets another jar of bees. She stings herself and within an hour or two she has more energy and is walking better. Some people do not feel like they are slipping backwards. They can miss 2-3 weeks and not notice any return of symptoms.

ISN'T BEE VENOM A POISON?

Like many medicines, bee venom does have toxic effects; all poison is a question of dosage. Many people take Cumadin to thin their blood, but in larger doses it is a rat poison. There is a famous story about an English doctor who is credited with discovering Digitalis. His name was Dr. Withering. In his time many people were dying from "dropsy," which is a heart condition. The doctors in London could not seem to find a remedy for this condition. One day Dr. Withering heard about a witch, who lived out in the country, who seemed to be helping people with dropsy. She was using a potion that contained the herb, foxglove, which is a poisonous plant. It also contains digoxin which strongly affects heart activity. With her help, Dr. Withering formulated the medication, Digitalis, which strengthens cardiac contraction and rate.

When Dr. Withering returned to London, the cardiac specialists condemned him and tried to bar him from practicing medicine. And yet now, he is credited with discovering Digitalis, a well-known and well-accepted drug for certain congestive heart problems.

As with all treatments, there are issues of toxicity and efficacy which affect therapeutic choice. Only time and clinical experience can tell.

WHAT IS THE CORRECT NUMBER OF BEE STINGS?

The correct number of bee stings for any one person is not really known. I recommend that you start with one, as a test sting, and then do several more on the first day. After that, you can work your way up slowly (perhaps increasing the number of stings by two at a time), until you hit 20 stings. Most people with a chronic condition seem to do well with 15-20, stings three times a week for about six months. If you are a very thin person, you may get by with fewer stings, and if you are more heavy set, you may want to do more stings. Listen to your body. It will tell you what you need and when you have gone too far.

IF BEE VENOM IS SO GREAT, WHY HAVEN'T THE MEDICAL DOCTORS AND SCIENTISTS SHOWN MORE INTEREST IN IT?

The answer to this question is plain and simple, as Charles Mraz says, "There's just no money in it!" It generally takes seven years and well over $100 million dollars to take a substance to market. A drug company cannot expect to cover this investment from a naturally occurring substance like bee venom. Further, live bee sting therapy does not easily lend itself to the double-blind controlled studies that scientists so dearly love. It is more likely, given the practicalities of medical politics, that any studies will use injectable venom, which is much less powerful than that of live bees. Such studies may be incomplete and the results inconclusive.

WHAT ARE THE RISKS OF DOING BEE VENOM THERAPY?

As described in the sections called "Reactions" and "Warnings," there are four kinds of allergic reactions to BVT—immediate systemic, delayed systemic, immediate localized, and delayed localized. An immediate systemic reaction, known as anaphylactic shock, occurs when the person has difficulty breathing—it is certainly a serious risk, but is exceedingly rare. Nonetheless, it is imperative that all bee venom therapists have a bee-sting kit on hand at all times, and know how to use it. This is also true if you are doing bee stings at home. You will need a bee-sting kit. You can get this by having your doctor write you a prescription for one. If you still have questions about this topic, please refer back to the sections titled "Reactions" and "Warnings."

HOW IS BEE VENOM COLLECTED?

Collecting bee venom is a long painstaking process. I have assisted Charlie Mraz in his collection of venom. He has been collecting it for 40 years. Every year he refines the process a little more. It can only be done in warm weather and you get the best results when the hives are very strong. First, you need a collecting board that will give the bees an electric shock. They will then sting the collecting board and deposit their venom under a rubber mat. Most of the bees will be able to separate themselves from the board and fly away without losing their stingers. You can only leave the collecting board on the hive for 10-15 minutes, brushing the bees off the board every few minutes so that other bees can go on it. But after the initial 10-15 minutes, the bees catch on to the situation and they will no longer sting the board. That's when you have to move it to another hive. The venom is then removed from behind the rubber mat and is dried. In order to reconstitute it back into an injectable form it is mixed with a saline solution. I believe this is why the injectable venom is not as potent as the real thing. When man tampers with Mother Nature, something is lost in the translation.

IS ALL INJECTABLE BEE VENOM THE SAME?

No, not all bee venom is created equal. Charlie Mraz's venom is considered to be the standard for venom in the US, according to the FDA. Everything else is measured against his venom. The venom from Europe and Asia is often polluted with feces, pollen and honey. There is also some very good venom coming out of Calgary, Canada (See Important Names and Addresses in Appendix II.)

HOW MANY BEES DOES IT TAKE TO MAKE ONE GRAM OF PURE BEE VENOM?

Charlie Mraz states that one gram of his dry venom is the product of approximately 10,000 bees. His "normal" bee venom solution is mixed in a ratio of 1 milligram of dry venom to 1 cc of isotonic solution. In this case, one tenth of a milliliter is equal to one bee sting. Obviously, all injectable bee venom will vary in strength based on the proportions of ingredients used.

Bee venom prepared for injection is approximately 1/20th the strength of one live bee sting. These injections can be useful for local ailments such as scars and relief of some chronic pain conditions such as phantom limb syndrome, low back pain, whiplash, sciatica. The live bees are much more effective, however, for treating systemic conditions, whether chronic or acute.

HOW CAN I FIND AN APITHERAPIST IN MY AREA?

Try contacting your local beekeeping association for a list of local beekeepers. Usually there is someone among the membership who does apitherapy. If you hit a dead end, call the American Apitherapy Association at

(800) 823-3460. They have a membership list of apitherapists that is available to those who join the society.

WHAT IS THE AMERICAN APITHERAPY SOCIETY (AAS)?

The AAS is a non-profit educational organization to which all donations are tax-deductible. The purpose of the AAS is to collect and distribute information on the subject of apitherapy. The AAS does not treat rather it serves as an information clearinghouse. It makes no claims about the risks or efficacy of apitherapy. If you wish to get more information, feel free to contact the AAS at P.O. Box 54, Route 12, Hartland Four Corners, VT 05049. Their telephone number is (800) 823-3460. You can support the AAS by competing and returning the feedback forms found in Appendix IV. You can also join the society.

HOW CAN I SUPPORT THE AMERICAN APITHERAPY SOCIETY?

You can support the AAS both clinically and financially. You can send in your data to the AAS so they can track your feedback. There is a feedback form in Appendix IV that you can send in. The more data they can collect, the better able they will be to serve us.

DID YOU KNOW THAT HONEYBEES HAVE BEEN MAKING HONEY FROM FLOWERS FOR 10–20 MILLION YEARS?

WHY DO HONEYBEES DIE WHEN THEY LOSE THEIR STINGERS?

The reason honeybees die after they sting a person is because the intestines of a female honeybee are attached to her stinger; so if she loses her stinger, she loses her intestines as well. She will eventually die within a day or two. The other honeybees will not let her back into the hive without a stinger, so she dies outside the hive. The stinger becomes detached and remains in the person's body until it is removed.

WHAT IS THE AVERAGE LIFE SPAN OF A HONEYBEE?

The average female worker honeybee lives approximately 4-8 weeks during the honey season. These worker bees literally wear their wings out collecting nectar and pollen and keeping the hive cool. They fan water droplets in the hive for air conditioning in the summer. The average drone (male honeybee which has no stinger) lasts 2-3 months during the same season. The queen bee usually lives 2-3 years, although I have heard of queens lasting up to 6 years.

HONEYBEES STROKE THEIR WINGS 11,400 TIMES EACH MINUTE . . . THAT'S WHERE THE BUZZING NOISE COMES FROM . . .

HOW MANY BEES ARE THERE IN A GOOD STRONG HIVE?

There are generally 30-40,000 honeybees in a strong hive in peak season. Approximately 500-1000 of those are drones, the rest are worker bees. There is usually one queen. Occasionally you will have two queens if the old one is about to die and a new one is produced.

HOW MANY MILES MIGHT A SINGLE BEE TRAVEL TO PRODUCE ENOUGH HONEY TO A ONE POUND JAR?

Bees may fly two or three miles to find the flower that has the right nectar to produce honey. An individual bee might travel as much as 40,000 miles to produce a one pound jar of honey.

THE AVERAGE SPEED OF A HONEYBEE IS 15 MILES PER HOUR. . .

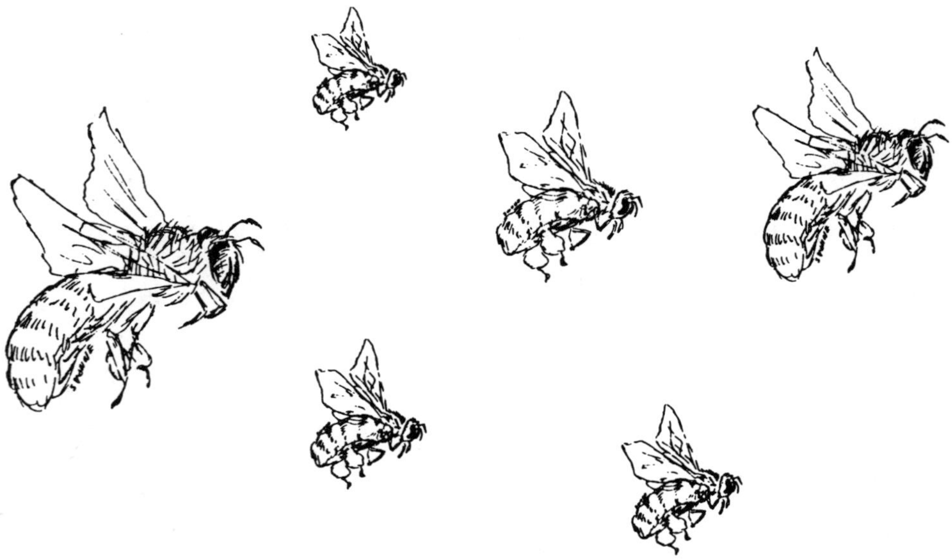

CHAPTER 2

"WHAT DO I NEED TO GET STARTED?"

Getting started is not difficult; just forget to be afraid and pull together the following materials:

FIRST YOU NEED A BEE STING KIT

You will need to have a bee sting kit (epinephrine and anti-histamine) available. You can get this kit by prescription from your doctor. Be sure you read the directions on the package before you get your test sting.

THEN YOU NEED BEES

For your initial stings, you'll probably just want to get bees already in a jar. Once you're sure you want to continue, you may want to enjoy the mysteries of having your own hive.

BEE'S TO GO

A good source for bees is your local beekeeper. Call your local có-op extension service or your state beekeeping association. Or, you can call Greg Ferris for bees by mail at (800) 787-HONY. When getting bees to go, make sure that the jar is prepared as described on the following page.

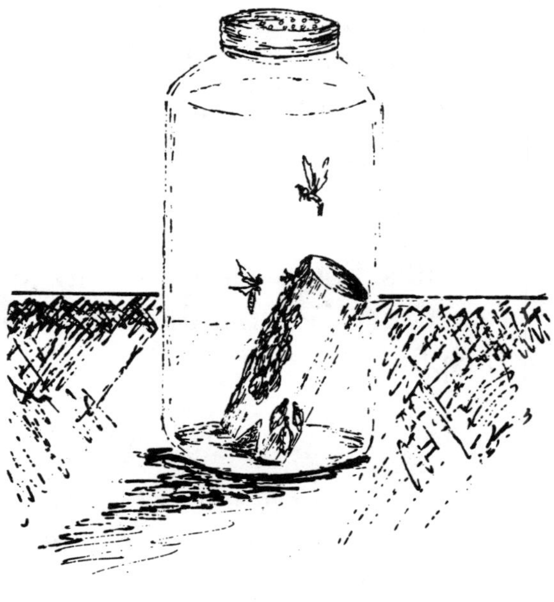

Bees-to-go

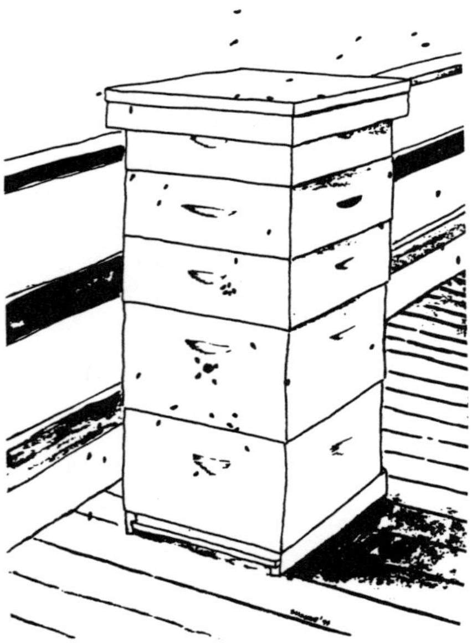

Get Your Own Hive

The following magazines are good sources for information about locating and keeping hives: "Bee Culture," A.I. Root Co., located at 623 West Liberty, Medina, OH 44256, and "The American Bee Journal," Dadant and Sons, Inc., 51 S. Second Street, Hamilton, IL 62341.

COLLECTING BEES FROM A HIVE

Here are some tips for getting bees out of a hive. Most hives have a large entrance on the bottom board on the front of the hive. Some people gather bees there. My preference is to collect bees through a hole drilled into one of the hive bodies. I actually have two holes in my hives. One is in the front of the hive, the other is in the back. I take a jar that is already prepared with honey, a tissue and a toilet paper roll, and remove the lid. Then I blow into the jar and place it up against the hole in the hive. Bees do not like the smell of animal breath, so they will come out of the hive to investigate the smell in the jar. I rattle the jar up against the side of the hive. The noise will upset them and they will continue to come out into the jar to find out what is going on. When I have enough bees, I slide the jar off to the side of the hive and quickly put the lid on tight.

Many people say they have trouble gathering bees in the cold winter months. Some beekeepers are afraid to open their hives at this time of year. They are concerned that they will disturb the hive. I have two suggestions that may be helpful:

- Place a piece of styrofoam insulation between the outside cover and the inner cover of the hive. It should be approximately the same size as the inner cover. Then spread honey or sugar water on the styrofoam board before the weather gets too cold. When the cold weather hits, bees will gather on the insulation board due to the warmth and the honey. When you need bees, lift up the outer cover and there will be plenty of bees on the styrofoam. You will be able to scrape them off the board and into your jar with a spoon.

↠ In the winter months I also warm the jars up with a hair dryer right before I place the jar against the hive. The bees love the warmth and they just pour right out of the hive and into the jar.

HOW TO KEEP BEES CALM AND ALIVE

Have bees in a jar with holes in the lid for air. Make sure you have enough honey (crystallized honey is best) and a tissue at the bottom of the jar. You also need a toilet paper roll or an index card for the bees to climb on. Cut two inverted V's at the bottom of the toilet paper roll. The bees also need water. Some people put in a one inch square sponge and soak it with water.

REMEMBER TO FEED YOUR BEES! If you use liquid honey, you will need to feed them a teaspoon of honey every day. A plastic honey bear, will help you squeeze the honey through the holes in the lid. If you use crystallized honey, you may only have to feed the bees every 5-7 days.

Once you get the bees in a jar there are several ways to calm them down. The calmer they are, the easier it is to get them out of the jar.

↠ Your bees will be calmer if you keep them stored in a dark place, like a closet. Keep them in a ventilated space; if you leave them in a closet, leave the door slightly ajar.

↠ You can put them in the freezer for five minutes. (Just don't forget about them!)

↠ You can spray them with water. (Don't overspray them or they will drown.)

PREPARING A JAR OF BEES FOR EXTENDED USE

Take a plastic jar and drill holes in the lid. Next take an ice pick and heat it. Then poke holes into the jar itself with the hot ice pick. Make two rows of holes all the way around the bottom of the jar, but not too low. Then make two rows of holes around the top of the jar. You can also make some holes along the side of the jar as well. These holes will give the bees plenty of fresh air to breathe.

To prepare the inside of the jar, do the following:

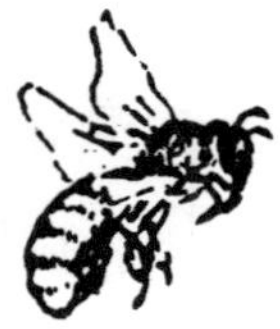

- Put a paper towel at the bottom of the jar.

- Place a empty toilet paper roll (with 2 inverted V's cut at the bottom of it) in the jar.

- Cut off the bottom of a styrofoam cup about one and one-half inches from the bottom. Place a few broken pieces of styrofoam in the bottom of this cup.

- Place half a piece of ice in the cup.

- Then cut a strip of honeycomb about 1 inch wide and 3 inches long. Lay it on a flat plate.

- Pour granulated sugar into the comb. Take a knife and spread the sugar onto all surfaces of the comb. Pack it in firmly. Make a heavy paste, so that the honey stays in the comb and doesn't run out. If you are unable to obtain honeycomb, you can put granulated sugar directly into liquid honey until you achieve a thick consistency.

- If the jar is very large and you are using more than one toilet paper roll, you will need one strip of honeycomb per toilet paper roll.

- To make sure the bees have enough water, you can also set a small ice chip on top of the jar over one of the holes. As it melts it will drip into the jar. If you position it correctly, you can actually get the ice to drip into the little styrofoam cup.

- Keep the jar in a dark place.

Some people have had success keeping the bees alive longer by letting them have a chance to fly out of the jar. After the bees have been in the jar for a couple of days, take them outside near a bush at dusk. Open the lid. The bees will fly out and defecate, which they won't do in the jar as it has become their hive. They will eventually return to the jar at night, because it has become their home. After it gets dark, go back and put the lid on the jar, and bring it inside. The bees will probably live longer if you use this technique.

PREPARING TO STING: CATCHING A BEE WITH TWEEZERS

It is helpful to be near a sunlit window while catching bees; if they get loose they will go to the light. With your tweezers, grasp a bee by the head or thorax, not the abdomen. It is helpful to use locking tweezers, or hemostats, which can be obtained at hobby stores as well as a medical supply house.

Consider placing ice on the area before and after you sting it. It is best not to put the ice on top of the stinger itself. You can, however, grasp the skin immediately around the stinger and squeeze it while the stinger is still in. Many people find that this reduces the pain.

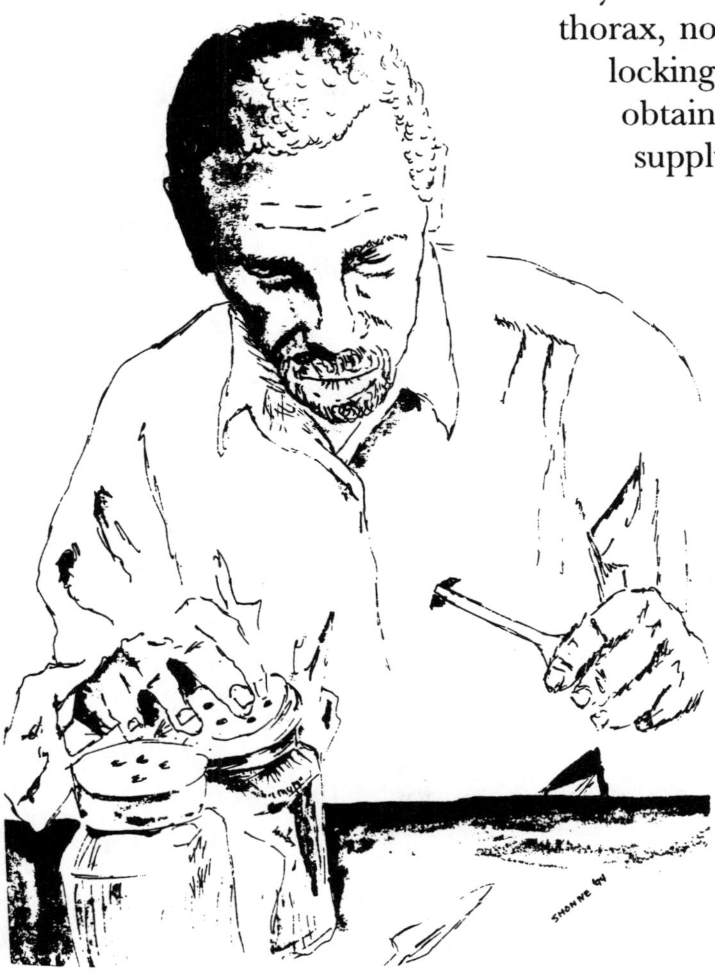

***Tweezey-does-it!** This is my friend Duke helping me catch bees in preparation for stinging.*

STINGING TECHNIQUE

Test Sting

Start with one test sting and take it out immediately. This is often done on the knee, because it is far away from the heart. Be sure to have your bee sting kit and know how to recognize the symptoms of an immediate generalized reaction (anaphylactic shock).

Initial Stings

If the person feels OK after 15-20 minutes, proceed with five more stings, usually on the low back. Remove the stingers 10-15 minutes later; take care to pull the stingers sideways along the skin and not straight up. It is best to stay away from the extremities (the arms and the legs) at first, because they tend to swell, especially in the beginning. Stinging on the trunk of the body tends to create less swelling in the beginning. The first month is the hardest. After a month or so, the redness, itching and swelling will diminish. This is normal and will make it easier to continue. After a while, your body will get used to the venom. Even though it will not react as much, the body will still get the effects of the venom.

If you don't want to leave the stinger in a long time due to a previously strong reaction, try not to squeeze the venom sac on top of the stinger while taking the stinger out, as this will squeeze out all the venom.

You can use Preparation-H or similar products such as a Benadryl cream or white vinegar, for soothing redness and itching. Ice can also be helpful. Some people find massaging the area around the sting site eases the pain. Remember, the bigger the reaction, the more potent the potential healing action. You may also experience a "healing crisis." If you experience flu-like symptoms or a feeling of fatigue, you may want to re-read the section on "Reactions," the discussion of "healing crisis" in Chapter 1, and Chapter 11, "What Do I Do If I Feel That I'm Not Getting Better."

Keep in mind that if you are taking medication, it may hinder the effectiveness of the bee stings. Consult you physician before making any change in your prescribed medications.

Progressive Stinging

It is important to increase the number of stings you get slowly. I usually start by giving six stings each of the first two sessions, then I go up to eight stings for two sessions, then ten stings, etc. In other words, I increase the number of stings by two each session. It is very important not to jump from eight stings to fourteen stings. Don't give the body more than it can handle too quickly or too early. Remember, "Slow and steady wins the race." You'll probably be doing bee stings for quite a while, so "take it easy." I have found working up to 15-20 stings per session is usually sufficient. While experienced apitherapists have been following this method for decades, some people are trying 6 to 8 stings a day, everyday. Use your own judgment, and see what works for you. But certainly, don't sting the same area over and over again. It is best to move around.

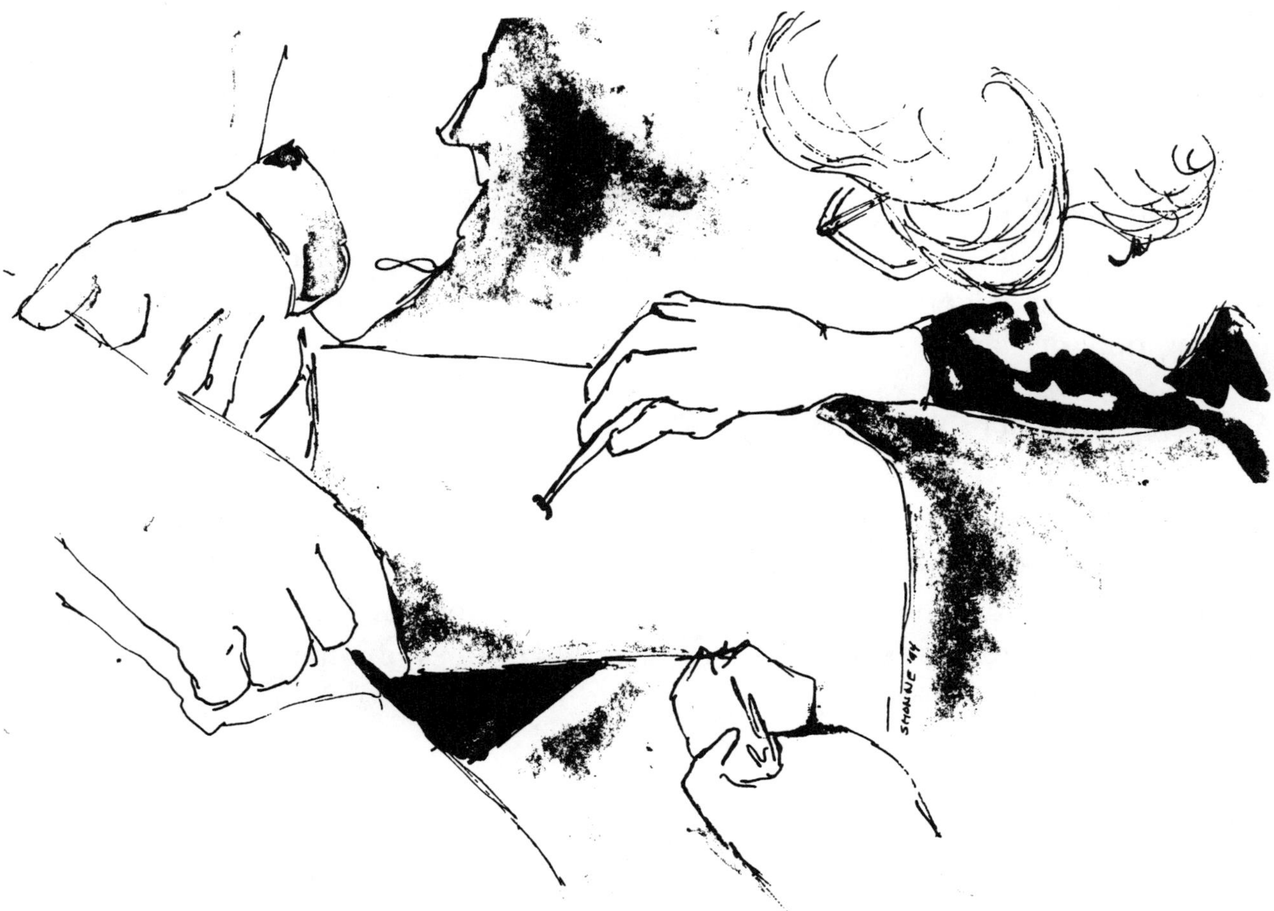

WHERE TO AIM

At the beginning, you will be stinging on "trigger points" and "nerve meridians." These will be fairly easy to locate. As described in Pat Wagner's instructions . . . sting where it hurts ("trigger points") and sting along the nerves as they come out of the spine, and down the legs and arms (like creases on a pair of pants and sleeves of a shirt). You may want to mark your spots with a felt tip pen. The following Chapter, "Where Do I Sting Myself?," describes the initial point selections in some detail. Part 2 teaches you how to make more advanced point selections based on Oriental acupuncture techniques.

A VACATION FROM BEES

If you have stopped the bee stings for more than two weeks for any reason, always start with one test sting. After 15 minutes you can proceed, but do not start at the level where you left off. Start with just a few stings and work your way up again.

TAKING A REST

Do not sting an area that is already red or swollen from the bee stings. It is important to give the body a rest. So if your leg is swollen or red, sting on the low back, the shoulders, or the spine. The idea is to move around. It's best not to sting only one area.

VITAMIN C ALERT

Be sure the person being stung knows that he needs 2-3000 milligrams of Vitamin C every day. Some people recommend as much as 6000 milligrams of Vitamin C for MS patients. This is an individual choice . . . but I wouldn't go below 2 or 3000 milligrams. If you are taking high does of Vitamin C and wish to quit, you should taper down over a period of days rather than simply quit.

BEE TENACIOUS

If you have a serious/chronic illness, it is recommended that you commit to doing the bee stings three times per week for at least six months. (If you are doing a lot better, you could possibly cut down to two sessions per week.)

Remember, it is important not to give up too early. You may be tempted to stop the bee stings if you don't notice changes right away. Please don't lose sight of the fact that you have a chronic illness. You didn't get this way overnight and this is not a magic pill that will get you well overnight. Healing is a process that takes time.

BEE CREATIVE: THE ORIENTAL WAY

Eventually you may want to try "bee-acupuncture," that is stinging yourself or others in acupuncture points. I do recommend that you stay with "trigger points" and "nerve meridians" for the first month or so. After your body has acclimated to the stings, you may want to branch out and benefit from the healing power of "bee-acupuncture." Once you have identified the points you want to sting, based on the work you will do later in this book, sting as close as you can relative to where you think the acupuncture point is on the chart. You may want to mark the spot with a pen first. The illustrations in this book are approximate to give you a rough idea. If you want, you can get another book on acupuncture that has the exact point locations written out in detail. This book is meant to give you a general idea where the points are. Don't worry about doing it "perfectly." There is room for a margin of error. If you were using needles, you would really need to be exact. But since you are using bee stings, the venom is going to spread out; you have a margin of error about the size of a nickel. Trust your intuition and remember that your intention when you sting yourself is as important as the location. Keep in mind your purpose, your goal. Keep your attitude positive. The only way to really be precise would be to go to an acupuncturist and have her mark you out.

"TO THE POWERS THAT BEE!"

RAE CAROL'S STORY

For some time now, I have believed that all we need to heal and care for ourselves (physically, mentally, and spiritually) is within us. The challenge is finding the knowledge and using it appropriately.

My final diagnosis came after graduating from college, a marriage, and two healthy pregnancies (which gave me two beautiful daughters). It was not until I found myself dealing with a divorce, that my MS showed its ugly face. Talk about choices! I was now faced with yet another challenge, another choice. What was the best way to deal with this diagnosis? I would not succumb to the disease! After all, I have MS, it doesn't have me! I don't like drugs and chemicals as a treatment for symptoms. When I have a headache, I try to deal with the problem causing the headache as opposed to popping two pills.

I had been researching possible ways to deal with my diagnosis of MS for quite a while, when my dear Grandmother, Mimi, first saw a local news program on Bee Venom Therapy. I spoke to Pat Wagner, "the Bee Lady" for over a year before I was finally ready to take the step. This was a step that I had discussed with my neurologist, who thought that there could very possibly "bee" MEDICINAL value in honeybee venom. No promises were made, but none were made using prednisone or solumedrol.

So my choice became clear: BVT, meditation, and nutrition. This was a holistic approach. Everything was working together as part of my balancing act. Out to Waldorf, MD to see Pat Wagner, I was driven by a friend, Jim Avery, who has shared many life experiences with me. As he aided me up the driveway, I remember thinking, "Bees? . . . Stings! . . . OH MY GOD!"

Well, 8 stings later, I realized I had arrived. Well into my third week I experienced what is known as a "healing crisis." I had prepared for this and knew it was coming. The day that it happened I had received 14 stings. I had gone to lunch, gone shopping and picked up my daughter from camp. I began to feel sick to my stomach and had some cramps. I was on my way to another mall, when I decided that I better go home.

Upon arriving home, I rushed to the bathroom. As I sat there in vain, I decided I needed to lie down. I rolled back and forth in pain on the bed. By now I had a temperature, but I was not afraid. I knew something good was happening, but my mother still called down to Waldorf. She was told that what was happening to me was, "Great, this is what we want to happen!" I think I finally fell asleep about 1 a.m. When I awoke, I felt incredibly good. I got up, had my hair and nails done, took my daughters shopping, had lunch, went to a wedding and reception, and really didn't feel like leaving at 11:30 p.m. Talk about the powers that bee!

I was a little scared to get 14 stings again, and it was the July 4th weekend and Pat was not stinging, so I stopped by Amber Rose's house. I could only bear two stings. That was my limit. The next time I went to Pat's house I walked down the driveway alone, without my cane! When I realized what I had done, I excitedly went back inside to tell everyone! From this point on, I continued with BVT every Monday, Wednesday and Friday. For a while I traveled to Waldorf to get my stings. Then I started going to Amber's home in August. Sometimes I just get "bees to go" and sting myself at home.

BVT has allowed me to maintain independence, mobility, to work full-time, to have phenomenal energy, and to take care of my children. It has given me an opportunity to maintain a full life, filled with endless possibilities. At one point I began to slack off my stings, thinking I was doing so well. "I don't need this," I thought to myself. "Wrong!" Let's say, at least for now, I really do need the bee stings. I still feel every sting. It does not feel good, but I'll gladly take seconds of pain for hours of pleasure! My neurologist is quite pleased with my stability, progress, and energy.

I want deeply to thank Charlie Mraz, Pat Wagner, and Amber Rose, and ALL THE POWERS THAT BEE for aiding in my balancing act . . . for beeing one of the missing pieces of my puzzle . . . for where in the world would I "BEE" without you!

RAE CAROL IS A VERY SPECIAL LADY. SHE IS A WONDERFUL MOTHER AND A VERY POSITIVE ROLE MODEL FOR HER CHILDREN. SHE REMINDS ME THAT YOU CAN DO ANYTHING YOU PUT YOUR MIND TO. A.R.

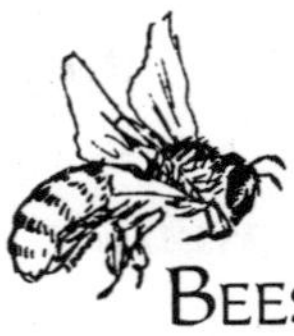

Bees seem to us to be thousands of individuals; it is more accurate to think of the hive as a single individual with thousands of individual cells.

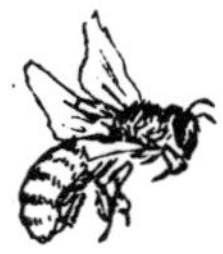

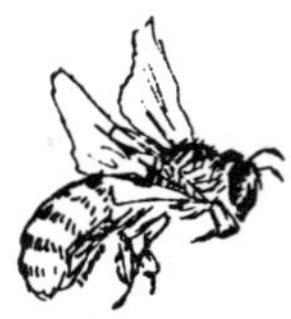

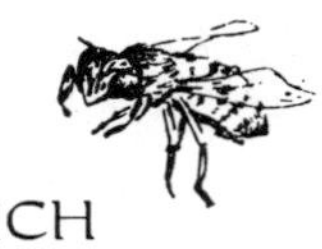

When a single bee dies, it is not a distinct life which perishes, but rather the loss of one cell to a organism still buzzing with life!

CHAPTER 3

"WHERE DO I STING MYSELF?"

There are five basic places to sting yourself or others:

"Trigger Points" or "Hot Spots"—These are points where it hurts! They vary from person to person, and from one day to the next. The Chinese call these "Ah Shi" points.

"Nerve Meridians"—These refer to nerve pathways that exit the spine and come down the arms and the legs. (See page 31.)

Acupuncture Pathways—The Chinese believe that energy or Ch'i flows through pathways in the body. These pathways are not nerves. If you cut the body open, you will not see them.

Acupuncture Points—Specific points on the acupuncture pathways are used to gain entrance to the vital energy. Acupuncture points are to acupuncture pathways like entrances and exits are to any major highway.

Scars—Any scars may block energy in the body. This is true even if the scar has been there a long time, or if you feel no discomfort from the scar. Scars from significant trauma, surgery, in important anatomical areas, or on pathways are good points to be treated.

"WHAT POINTS DO I USE FIRST?"

These instructions are for the first two-four weeks.

After you've successfully completed your test sting, go to the trunk of the body and do five more stings. If you have bladder problems, you may want to start with Pat Wagner's bladder points (See page 34). Use "trigger points" and "nerve meridians" on the back for the arms and legs. You can treat your legs by stinging the lower back and sacral area. Stinging the shoulders will help the arms and hands. If you go directly to the arms and legs too soon, you may swell a great deal. If you have any scars on the trunk of your body, it would be very beneficial to sting the scar itself or right next to it.

After a week or two, you can branch out to the arms and legs. Initially, sting just the upper arms and thighs. When working with the arms, imagine a shirt. Visualize the creases and sting along them. To sting points for the thighs, follow seams and creases on an imaginary pair of pants.

Eventually, over time, work your way down past the elbow and knee creases. I don't sting the forearms and calves until the person can handle the itching and swelling on their upper arms and thighs. Remember, to sting any scars you have on the arms and legs.

For the first month, I recommend you use the following instructions, provided courtesy of Pat Wagner. These instructions use "trigger points" and "nerve meridians" related to various illnesses or symptoms; these have primarily been developed as a response to MS, but can be used or adapted for a wide variety of ailments. After a month or so, you may want to explore a variety of acupuncture pathways and points. It is also important to note that if a scar cuts across an acupuncture pathway, it may block the flow of energy. In this case, you would sting the closest acupuncture points above and below the scar on that pathway.

IF YOU HAVE A SERIOUS ILLNESS, YOU MUST BE PREPARED TO COMMIT TO THIS THERAPY FOR AT LEAST SIX MONTHS, PREFERABLY THREE TIMES A WEEK! You may be able to cut down to twice a week as you start to feel better.

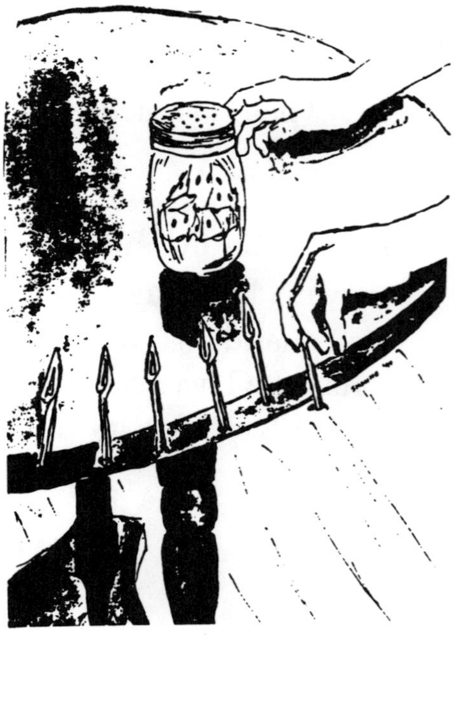

Lined up and ready to go!

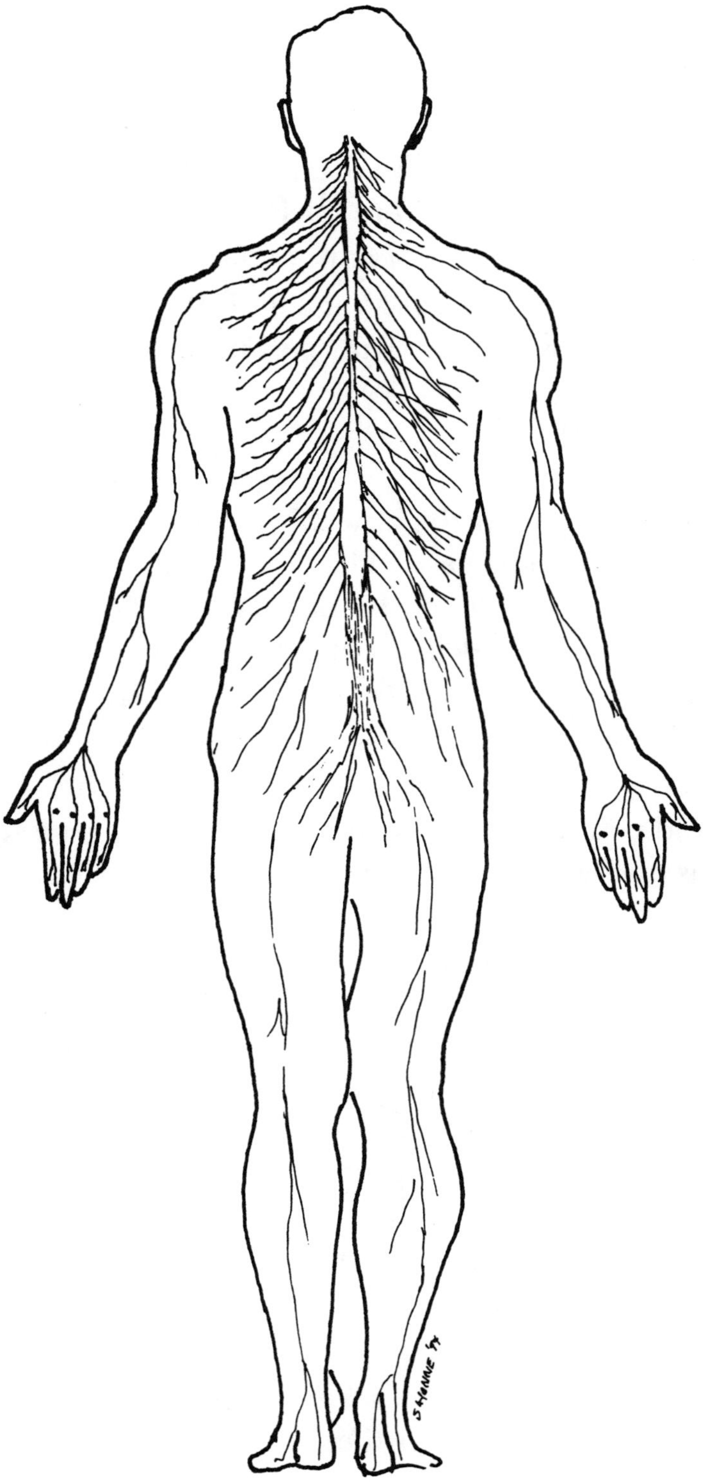

"Nerve Meridians"—*This drawing gives you an idea of the location of the major nerve pathways. Note that these pathways come out of the spine, and that they also travel down the arms and legs like the creases and seams in a shirt and a pair of pants.*

PAT'S SPECIFIC BEE STING SUGGESTIONS

From
HONEYBEE HEALING
(a.k.a. APITHERAPY)
"apis" is Latin for bees

FOR MULTIPLE SCLEROSIS

When starting bee venom therapy (BVT), plan to continue for at least 6 months, then on an as-needed basis. Plan on 3 sting sessions each week. For example, you might sting yourself on Monday, Wednesday and Friday. Start with 6-14 stings the first two sessions, depending on the severity of your symptoms and your weight. Increase by 4 stings for the next 2 or 3 sessions, and so on—reaching a maximum of 20-40 stings at each session, *as needed.* Men seem to respond best with more stings than women need. Sorry guys, but you can take it. Remember, you're tough! Should you reach a plateau in your healing process, increase by 10 stings for 2 sessions and then drop back to your previous level of stings.

FOR YOUR FEET AND LEGS

Get six stings in the lumbar region (low back, below waist level). Beginning at the bottom of the spine (backbone), get one sting on each side. Then, moving up about two inches, sting each side again. Repeat this once more, totalling 3 stings on each side. (That's 6). Now, on each of your buttocks, give 3 stings in the shape of a triangle with the point down. (That's 6 more). Next session, sting 3 times on the outside of each hip, 3 on the outside of each thigh (high, middle, and low) and one on the inside of your thigh (middle). Congratulations! That was 14.

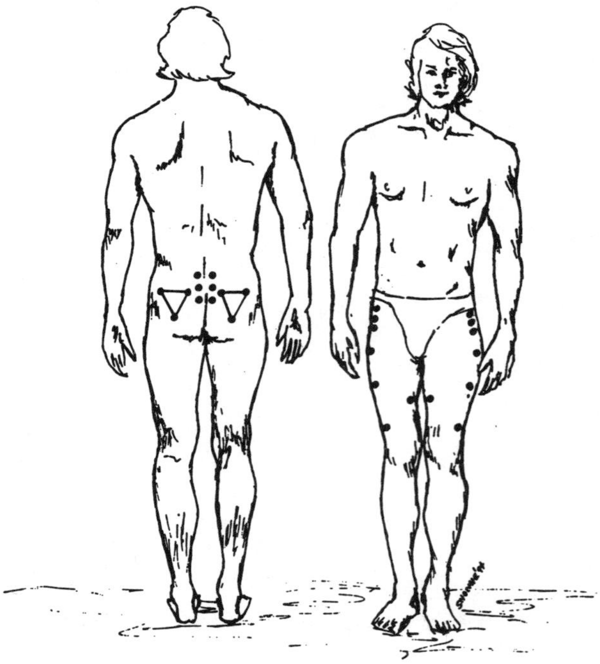

For another session you can sting directly on your lower back and spine and find and sting sore spots on your feet and ankles.

FOR YOUR HANDS AND ARMS

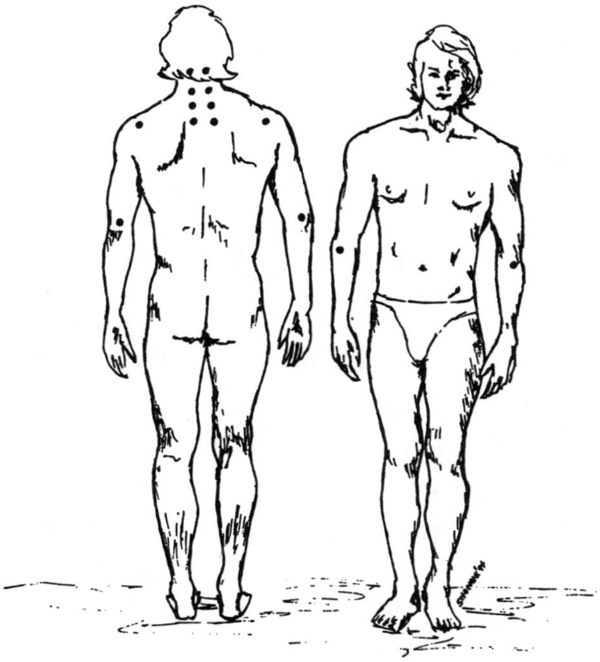

Start with a sting on each side of the spine (backbone) at the shoulder-blade level. Next, get stung on the back of your shoulder where your arm joins your body. Now, get a sting on each elbow and then each forearm, about an inch below the elbow. The second sting session, get 2 stings on each side of the back of your neck (about 2 inches apart vertically) and one sting about 2 inches below each of the neck stings (on your upper back/shoulder). As you increase the number of stings, continue in the same general areas, being sure to move down the forearm a bit, while stinging the elbow itself, the shoulder joint, the spine, etc.

FOR BALANCE

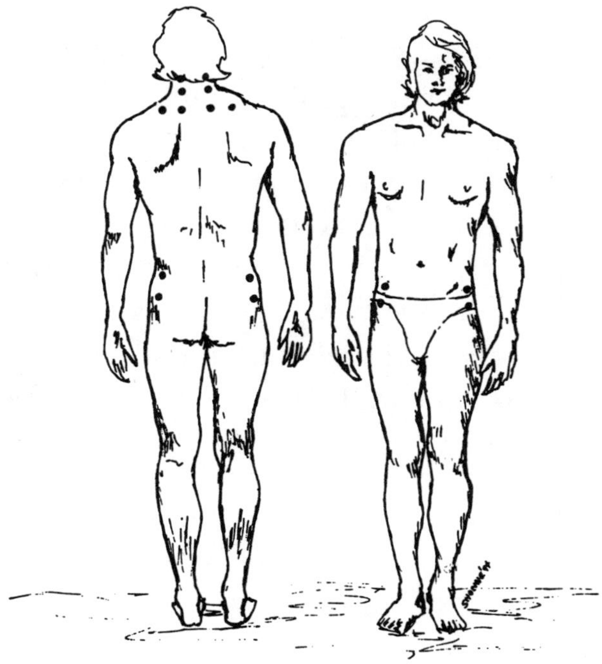

Sting the neck and high back/shoulder muscle as you would for the second session for your hands and arms. Also, sting your hips—front and back and sting high and low on the hip bone. If you have trouble wriggling your toes, get stung quite low on the outside of your shin bone. Make sure your toes can grasp. This is important for balance. Any or all of these areas could be causing your balance problems.

FOR FOOT DROP

To lift your foot but keep your heel on the ground, now and then get stung low on the back of your lower leg above the ankle level.

FOR TOE DRAG

Sting low on the outside of your shin bone as often as necessary.

FOR BLADDER PROBLEMS

To fight infection and/or to have better bladder control, get 2 stings just below the top of the pubic hair, left and right of center about 1 to 2 inches apart. Do this 3 times each week. Most people notice improvement in bladder control in about 2 weeks.

FOR BOWEL PROBLEMS

Stings in general, but especially in the low-back area, often seem to improve this problem. Eating raw honey is very good for the digestive system as well as muscle relaxation and, therefore, also seems to help with bowel problems. In addition, when the problem exists, men have said they found lumbar stings helped to improve their sexual functioning ability.

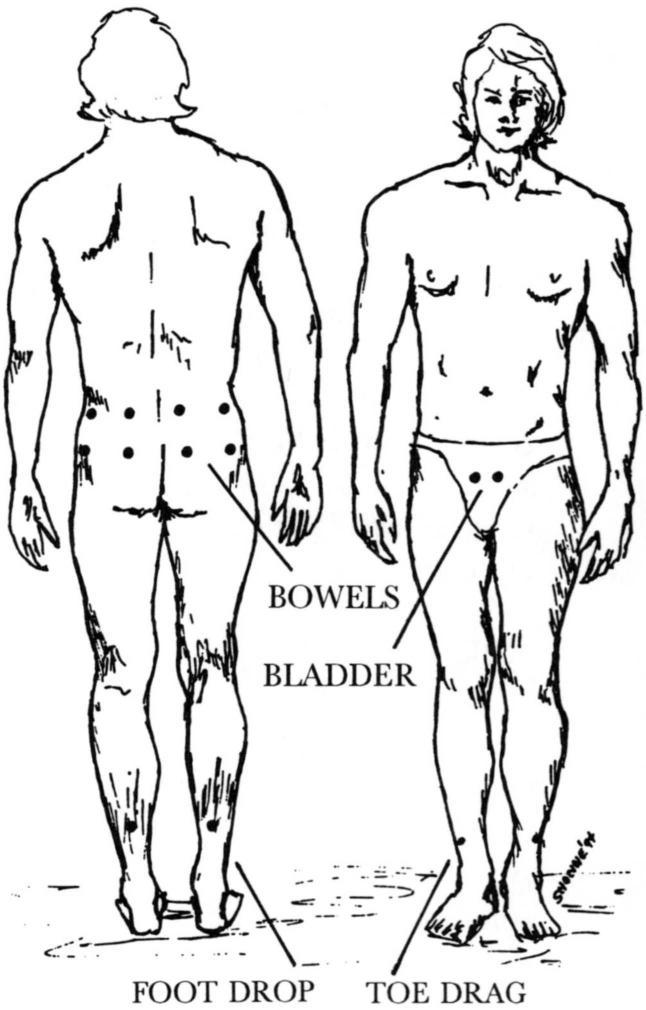

FOR VISION AND HEARING PROBLEMS

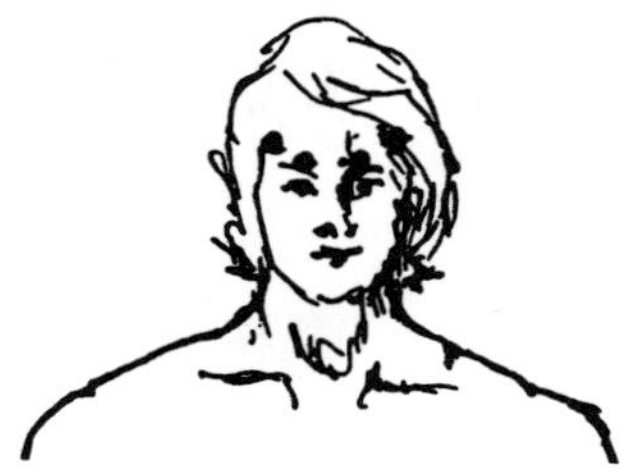

Stings on the back of the head (about 1 inch from the base of the skull) left and right of center, straight down from there on the neck at the base of the skull, and about 1 inch down from there on the neck can help with both vision and hearing difficulties. Stings in the temples and on the eyebrows can help too. These "head shots" do hurt, so use ice right on the stingers.

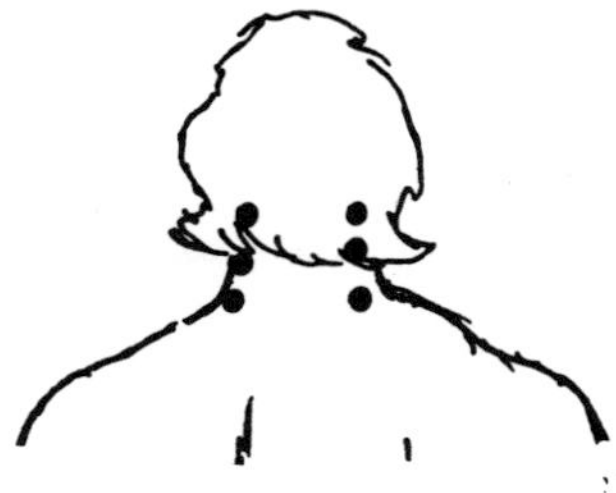

OTHER RELATED MS PROBLEMS

Bee stings work systemically. Once you have acquired a good saturation of bee venom in your system through getting stings—about 2 to 3 weeks—most people seem to feel a "sense of well being." You will most likely find you are less prone to colds, flu, further exacerbations, etc. When your immune system is working more properly, you should feel better. Also, do you do things such as walk into a room and forget why you went in there? I call that "fuzzy thinking." You will find that bee venom can, systemically, take care of that too. Look for other changes. Although vision and hearing problems can improve, NEVER STING THE EYEBALL OR INSIDE THE EAR. Just about everywhere else is fine.

FOR ARTHRITIS, GOUT, ETC.

Sting where it hurts! Several sting sessions as needed should be all it takes. Expect some swelling and then a decrease or elimination of arthritis pain.

FOR PMS, IRREGULAR MENSTRUAL CYCLES, ETC.

Two low-back stings twice a week for 4 to 6 weeks should be all it takes.

ONE MORE THING:

PLEASE REMEMBER TO THANK GOD FOR THE HONEYBEES!

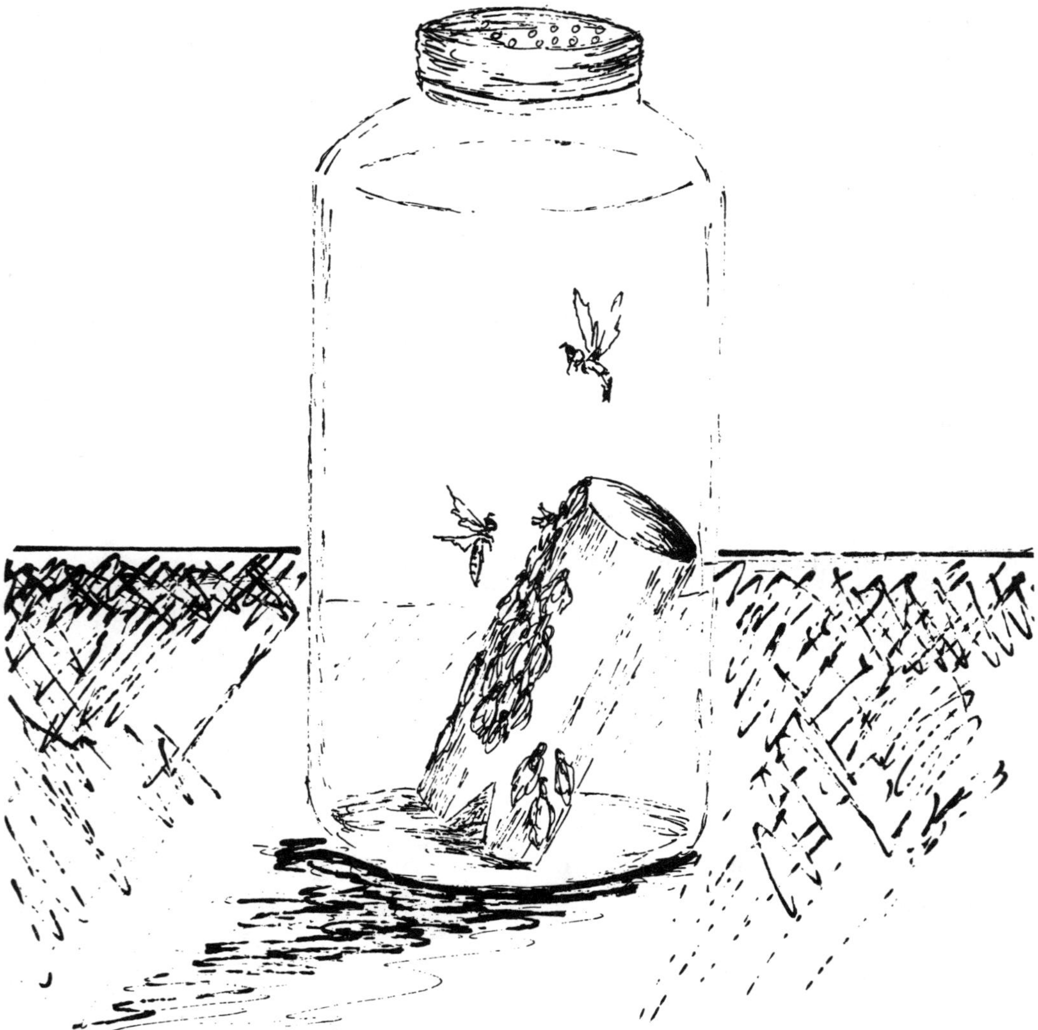

"THE ENERGY IS UNBELIEVABLE!"

TOM'S STORY

I am a 46 year old white male. I was diagnosed with MS in January of 1985. I went quickly from one cane to two canes, to a walker, to a wheelchair, and then to a three-wheeled scooter. In January of 1993, I had seriously considered retiring on a disability from my job as a librarian in a public high school. The major problem was the overwhelming fatigue that made the job almost impossible. I was sleeping twelve to fourteen hours a night, plus naps in the afternoon. I would be going to bed at eight/nine o'clock at night. It was not unusual for me to catch myself falling asleep as I drove down the road!

In June of 1993, my wife persuaded me to see a lady in southern Maryland, Pat Wagner, who was using Bee Venom Therapy with MS patients. It was there that I had the good fortune to meet Amber Rose, who was starting to offer this therapy at her house, which was much closer to me. I started receiving bee stings in July and over the next ten months worked my way up to 75 stings a week. During this time, Amber was a guide and mentor. She did much to ease my misgivings and educate me at the same time. At the present time I'm receiving 35 stings a week. The following changes I directly attribute to the bee venom.

1. The fatigue is almost totally gone. I sleep approximately 4 to 6 hours a night instead of 12 to 14 hours. I don't take naps anymore, and I have not wrecked the van.

2. When I started the bee stings my legs were very numb, very cold to the touch, and very white. Now, my legs are very sensitive to touch, very warm, and rosy in color. Also, the hair on my legs had disappeared with the MS and now, after the bee stings, it's starting to grow back!

I must admit that I was very skeptical about this treatment when I started. I didn't realize how rooted I was in Western medicine. But being told that there was no remedy or medicine that would mitigate the MS started me looking in other directions.

TOM IS A JOY TO WORK WITH . . . A.R.

DID YOU KNOW THAT THE PATRON SAINT FOR BEEKEEPING IS ST. AMBROSE?

CHAPTER 4

WE ARE ALL DOROTHYS AND TOTOS, AND WE ARE JUST TRYING TO FIND OUR WAY HOME

When I was 12 years old I played Dorothy in "The Wizard of Oz" at a local community center. As many of you may remember, Dorothy and her dog Toto were transported by a tornado to a far away land. The rest of the story is about how they try to find their way home again.

In the final scene, Dorothy clicks her ruby red slippers together and says over and over again, "There's no place like home! There's no place like home!" I believe that all sickness is really "homesickness;" we are all just trying to find our way home again, just like Dorothy and Toto.

If I win the lottery today, then I will have no desire to go back to yesterday. But if I get a diagnosis of cancer, MS, or AIDS today . . . I may yearn for yesterday . . . I may want to go back to a time when everything was OK and I felt safe. Just like the old Beatles song says, "Yesterday, all my troubles seemed so far away, now it looks as though they're here to stay, oh, I believe in yesterday." I believe that all of us just want to go back "home" to a time and a place when we were OK, before we were knocked off balance. We are feeling lost and we so desperately need the directions to find our way home, back to our center.

I would like to share with you a quotation from a book called "All Sickness is Homesickness" by Dianne Connelly (one of my acupuncture teachers):

> In a days time I am lost and found over and over again. Forgetting and recalling myself over and over again. The kingdom of illness is designed on a pattern of forgetting, a forgetting that has gotten stuck, a forgetting that seems to have no remembering, a forgetting that would have us be lost to ourselves, a forgetfulness of being. So, if I take you to my forgetting, to my sickness, and you bring yourself as guide, as coach, as practitioner, once more I come home, and see that I have been home all along, and that my illness

has been instrumental in leading me there one more time. I interpret the everlasting comings and goings of the dance called life, the alternating forgettings and rememberings, the endless agonies and ecstacies of daily life . . . . The story of the Taoist farmer illustrates a way of interpreting the dance of life's events:

> The farmer's horse ran away. That evening the neighbors gathered to commiserate with him, since this was such bad luck. He said, "Maybe." The next day the horse returned, but brought with it six wild horses, and the neighbors came exclaiming at his good fortune. He said, "Maybe." And then, the following day, his son tried to saddle and ride one of the wild horses, was thrown and broke his leg. Again, the neighbors came to offer their sympathy for his misfortune. He said, "Maybe." The day after that, the conscription officers came to the village to seize young men for the army, but because of the broken leg the farmer's son was rejected. When the neighbors came to say how fortunately everything had turned out, he said, "Maybe."
>
> Lieu Tze, as told by Alan Watts

Home is all embracing, a continuous inclusion of all events: this too and this too and this too. Home is en route. Home is the place from which we come and to which we return, Home is where I always am. All circumstances call me to new steps in the dance. All sickness points me there. All sickness is homesickness. All healing is homecoming. Sharing moves me homeward.

"All Sickness is Homesickness" by Dianne Connelly, 1993, pages 24-25.

This book is my effort to help you find your way home. May it be a new pair of glasses through which you see the world, a new set of directions, if you will, on your road map as you journey back toward health.

We are all Dorothys and Totos, and we are just trying to find our way home again. You may be lost now, but remember, you're on your way home. There is nothing wrong with asking for directions if you are lost . . . and you never know, maybe someday you'll be guiding others. Good luck. May God bless you on your journey homeward.

PART 2

ORIENTAL MEDICINE

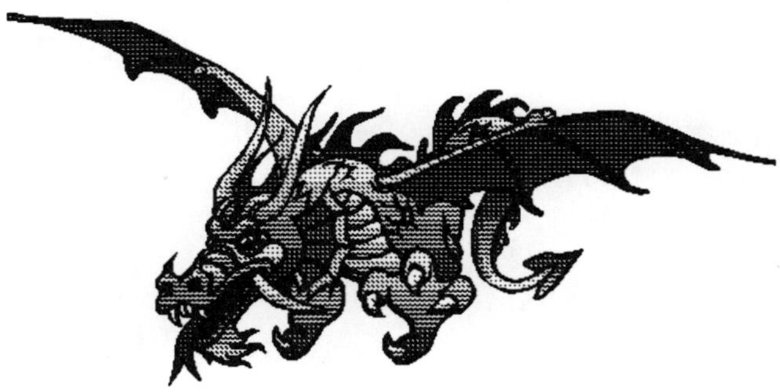

CHAPTER 5

THE PHILOSOPHY OF ORIENTAL MEDICINE: THE BASIC LAWS OF ACUPUNCTURE

All true healing comes from nature. Five thousand years ago, the ancient Chinese believed that the world was made up of five basic elements: wood, fire, earth, metal and water. These correspond to the seasons of the year and the seasons within us. Each of us was knocked off balance somewhere in childhood on one of these elements and never quite recovered.

The ancient Chinese developed acupuncture as a method of bringing the body back into balance. They believed that all sickness was due to an imbalance in the body, mind and spirit. Their basic goal was to restore balance and maintain harmony. They did this by removing blocks that prevent the free flow of energy in the body. Then the body heals itself. Traditional acupuncture treats the whole person, not just the symptoms.

According to ancient oriental philosophy, every human being is part of nature. Each one of us is a miniature cosmos, a replica of the great cosmos (that is nature). We are each unique in our own way and yet we are the same. Just like snowflakes, no two are exactly the same and yet they are all snowflakes.

There is an order to nature, but within that order, nature is in a state of constant flux. It is in accordance with this principle that our world is always changing. Nature does her dance, she is our teacher. Nature has her patterns, yet we cannot count on anything to remain the same.

Ancient wisdom says, "Change is the only truth in the universe" and "there is nothing permanent but change." The weather changes, the seasons change, and so, we too, must be open to change. When we stop growing or we resist change, we are more likely to get sick. We must keep our bodies in a relaxed and open state to keep energy flowing. We must follow the way of the Tao. Tao refers to the whole of life, and your path within it.

PATHWAYS AND THE FLOW OF CH'I

Acupuncture is a branch of Oriental Medicine which assists the healing process by using needles to either stimulate (tonify) or calm (sedate) specific points along pathways of energy which are called meridians. These meridians are not anatomically distinct, but have been discovered by the Chinese through centuries of experience and a sensitivity to the flow of life energy. This energy flows through this series of channels in an orderly flow that assists the body in maintaining harmony.

There are 12 major meridians which are bilateral, meaning that they flow along both sides of the body. The location of the pathway and its points is symmetrical. This book also describes points on two extra meridians, which are found at the front and rear center line of the body and are not bilateral.

The Chinese discovered that illness in the body, mind, or spirit is often accompanied by blocks in the flow of this energy. These blocks can be alleviated in many circumstances by using needles to "direct" the energy in a way that restores the smooth flow of energy. Acupuncturists also use a technique called Moxibustion, in which heat is added to the point.

The energy of the life force we are talking about is called "*Ch'i*" or "Qi" by the Chinese. This energy flows through the meridians. The Chinese character for *Ch'i* is a cooking vessel filled with rice. Steam is coming out of it. The *Ch'i* is not even the steam but the essence of the steam. *Ch'i* is considered to be totally non-physical.

The points along the meridians are openings into the flow of *Ch'i* which allow a needle, or a honeybee sting, to affect the quality of *Ch'i* in the meridian. This is where you can gain access to the person. Each point has its own unique function or "spirit." The art of acupuncture is to determine the changes in energy flow needed and what points to use to bring about those changes.

This is done first by a series of cleansings to clear blockages, by balancing treatments on the element(s) most out of balance, and then by using seasonal points and "spirit points." The names of certain acupuncture points (Spirit Burial Ground, Greater Mountain Stream, Spirit Path, and Joining the Valleys) call forth a need to return to the earth, while other points (Windows of the Sky[G], Soul

Door, and Utmost Source) speak to our yearning to reach for the sky and touch the stars.

Each person is given the opportunity for a personal vision quest through acupuncture, so that they may experience the alchemy of turning their suffering into gold.

YIN/YANG

In oriental philosophy the principle that the world is always changing is known as the Law of Yin/Yang. Life takes place in the alternating rhythm of yin and yang. There is a continual interchange and communication between the two. Day gives way to night and night to day. There is a cold, dark side of the mountain (yin) and a warm, sunny side of the mountain (yang). Everything has an inside (yin) and an outside (yang), a top (yang) and a bottom (yin). Flowers open (yang) and close (yin).

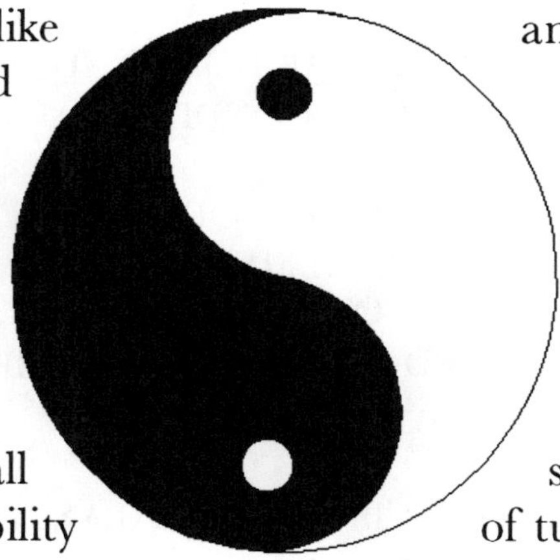

Yin and yang are like an inseparable couple. Their proper and balanced relationship is health, while a disturbance in their relationship is dis-ease. If you look at the yin/yang symbol you will see a small black dot within the white area. This is the yin within the yang. The small white dot within the black area is the yang within the yin. Nothing is pure yin or pure yang. Each has a small seed of the other. Everything has the possibility of turning into its opposite.

THE LAW OF THE FIVE ELEMENTS

A central understanding in the Chinese view of healing flows directly from the yin/yang principle. The tension between yin and yang creates five phases or elements. The Chinese saw the world as composed of WOOD, FIRE, EARTH, METAL (AIR), AND WATER. These elements follow the order of the five seasons of nature: SPRING, SUMMER, LATE SUMMER, AUTUMN, AND WINTER.

The five elements are as different from each other as five different notes on a scale. Therefore, the five seasons have five different qualities. Spring is very different from autumn and summer is nothing like winter. Each of the five elements has correspondences that go with it. Each element has a color, a season, a taste, an odor, a sound, an organ, a time of day, etc., associated with it. (Please see corresponding chart.)

Each element also has an emotion associated with it. Anger (the emotion that goes with the spring and the wood element), feels very different than joy (the emotion that goes with the summer and the fire element). So, as you can see, each element is distinctly different from the other elements. But each one has an affect on the others. In brief, people who have a particular element out of balance will feel the following:

> WHEN THE WOOD ELEMENT IS OUT OF BALANCE, THE PERSON MAY FEEL ANGRY, FRUSTRATED, IMPATIENT AND CONFUSED. THIS PERSON NEEDS A PLAN, A SENSE OF DIRECTION, AND HOPE.
>
> WHEN THE FIRE ELEMENT IS OUT OF BALANCE, THE PERSON MAY BE DEPRESSED, LACK JOY, OR APPEAR COLD AND DISTANT. THIS KIND OF PERSON NEEDS WARMTH, UNCONDITIONAL LOVE, AND JOY.
>
> WHEN THE EARTH ELEMENT IS OUT OF BALANCE, THE PERSON MAY WORRY A LOT OR HAVE A NEED TO TAKE CARE OF OTHERS (PERHAPS ALWAYS PUTTING OTHERS BEFORE THEMSELVES). THIS PERSON IS GOING TO NEED COMPASSION, SYMPATHY, AND TO BE UNDERSTOOD.
>
> WHEN THE METAL ELEMENT IS OUT OF BALANCE, THE PERSON MAY BE STUCK IN GUILT, GRIEF, LOSS, EMPTINESS, OR NEGATIVE THINKING. THIS TYPE OF PATIENT NEEDS TO BE RESPECTED, APPRECIATED, AND TO FEEL THAT LIFE HAS MEANING.
>
> WHEN THE WATER ELEMENT IS OUT OF BALANCE, THE PATIENT MAY HAVE A GREAT DEAL OF FEAR. THIS PERSON NEEDS REASSURANCE THAT EVERYTHING IS GOING TO BE O.K. THE PERSON NEEDS TO FEEL POWERFUL AND COURAGEOUS.

FIVE ELEMENT CORRESPONDENCES

TOPIC:	WOOD	FIRE	EARTH	METAL	WATER
Organ (function)	Gallbladder (decisionmaker) Liver (planner/architect)	Heart (supreme controller) Small Intestine (sorter) Heart Protector (joy, trust, sexuality) Three Heater (thermostat/networker)	Stomach (rotting & ripening) Spleen (energy transport)	Lungs (receives pure *Ch'i* from heavens) Colon (garbage collector)	Bladder (water storage) Kidney (water controller)
Time of Day	11 p.m.—3 a.m.	11 a.m.—3 p.m. 7 p.m.—11 p.m.	7 a.m.—11 a.m.	3 a.m.—7 a.m.	3 p.m.—7 p.m.
Color	green	red	yellow	white	blue
Season	spring	summer	late summer	autumn	winter
Taste	sour	bitter	sweet	spicy	salty
Odor	rancid	scorched	fragrant	rotten	putrid
Sound	shouting	laughing	singing	weeping	groaning
Emotion	anger	joy	sympathy	grief	fear
Orifice	eyes	ears	mouth	nose	two lower orifices
Sense Organ	eyes	tongue	lips	nose	ears
Fluid Secretion	tears	sweat	saliva (lips)	mucus	saliva (teeth)
Part of Body	ligaments/tendons	vessels	flesh	body hair	bones
External	nails	color of	lips	body hair	head hair
Climate	wind	heat	damp	dry	cold

Shen: The Cycle of Creation

Health and disease result from the quality and the flow of life energy. There are two major kinds of relationships (or cycles) within the five elements: the creation cycle and the control cycle. In the creation cycle, also called the Sheng or the Shen cycle, the energy flows from one meridian or pathway to the next in the order described in the accompanying Shen chart. The energy in this creation cycle flows in a clockwise direction around the circle. The flow is continuous. The cycle of energy has no beginning and no end. The five elements are inseparable. You can't have one without the others. Each element gives birth to the next one on the cycle. This brings us the Law of Mother and Son. Since one element gives birth to the next one on the cycle, wood is the mother of fire, and fire is the son of wood, and so on around the circle.

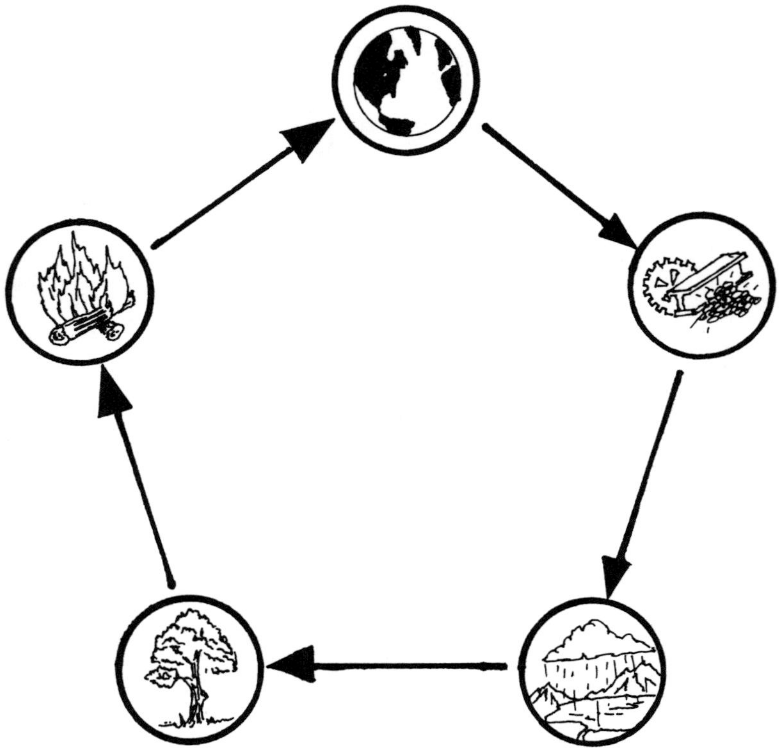

Shen Cycle: *This chart depicts the Shen cycle, or the cycle of creation, in which each element gives birth to the next one. Each element is the mother of the next. Understanding the clockwise flow and the order in which each element is the mother to the next is central to understanding this Law of the Five Elements.*

The flow of Shen can be thought of in this manner:

WOOD CREATES FIRE Two pieces of wood together can produce a spark.

FIRE CREATES EARTH Fire transforms burning matter into ashes.

EARTH CREATES METAL Within the earth, metal (ore) is buried.

METAL CREATES WATER Metal becomes a liquid when it melts.

WATER CREATES WOOD A tree cannot grow without water.

This concept becomes important for purposes of diagnosis, because sometimes the element that is the "child" has more symptoms than the "mother" element. Now, what this means in terms of dis-ease is that if the fire element is out of balance (or "sick") then the earth element will be struggling as well, because its getting either too much or too little energy from its mother, fire. In the Law of Mother and Son, we often notice that the son may cry out louder than the mother. When the fire element is out of balance, for example, you might get a lot of symptoms in the earth element. You may be tempted to treat the earth. If the real problem is that the fire element is out of balance, treating the earth element may only give you temporary relief. This is because you are treating the symptoms (the child) and not the root cause (the mother). On the other hand, let's say you have a lot of symptoms on the fire element. It's possible that the earth element is really the first one that went out of balance and you're getting symptoms in the fire element because it's the mother of the earth. In this case, treating the symptoms (fire), will be less successful than treating the root cause (the earth). The reason I am mentioning this is that if you decide to work on a certain element first and you don't get the desired results, you may want to treat the element either before it or after it on the five element cycle.

If a mother does not have enough milk or if she is too weak to take care of her child, the baby may start to cry. Let's say we hear the baby crying. So we go into the room and pick up the crying child. The child may stop crying for a while, but we must also help the mother. If we don't, then sooner or later, after we put the child down, it will begin to cry again. This is the best argument I know for not just treating symptoms. The cause of the symptoms may be coming from someplace else. You could end up chasing symptoms forever.

Going back to our analogy, we may need to support the mother and reconnect her with the child. Therefore, we may have to treat the fire element before we treat the earth element. I realize it may be very tempting to treat the earth element first, because it has more symptoms, but I strongly encourage you to try and identify the cause of the problem not just the symptoms. I will explain this in more detail as we go on.

The Mother/Son relationship does not go backwards, because the energy of the creation cycle only moves in a clockwise direction. For example, if a child is hungry, you bring the mother to the child and give him the mother's breast. This is assuming the mother is strong and there is enough milk. But if the mother is hungry or weak, you don't give her the child to eat. So, in other words the cycle does not go backwards; earth does not give to fire. This would be like the child taking care of the mother and that is not the way it is supposed to be. That is out of balance. That would be a dysfunctional family; as a mother should not have a son in order to be loved, so the element which is the "son" cannot take care of the "mother."

K'o Cycle: The Dance of Control

This energy brings us to the second kind of relationship within the five elements. The K'o or control cycle. The balance of energy in the body is maintained not only by Shen's creating and feeding the next element, but by K'o's limitation of the energy through control. Water is the mother of wood and wood is the mother of fire; therefore water is the grandmother of fire. This relationship of checks and balances is called the K'o cycle and this feedback cycle helps keep the *Ch'i* in balance. The grandmother controls the grandchild by her presence, just by being there. For example, the presence of water holds fire in check. If there is too much water, it will put out the fire. Water, which is the grandmother of the fire, will keep excessive fire in balance. This is not a flow of energy like the creation cycle. It is not feeding the fire; but regulating its intensity.

This control can become destructive if it becomes overbearing. When the K'o cycle is in a state of imbalance it becomes a destructive cycle:

WOOD DESTROYS EARTH The tree begins to suck strength from the earth

EARTH DESTROYS WATER Earth can halt the flow of water (like a dam)
Earth can soak up too much water (like a mud slide)

WATER DESTROYS FIRE Water will extinguish or put out the flame

FIRE DESTROYS METAL Fire will cause metal to melt

METAL DESTROYS WOOD The axe can cut down the tree

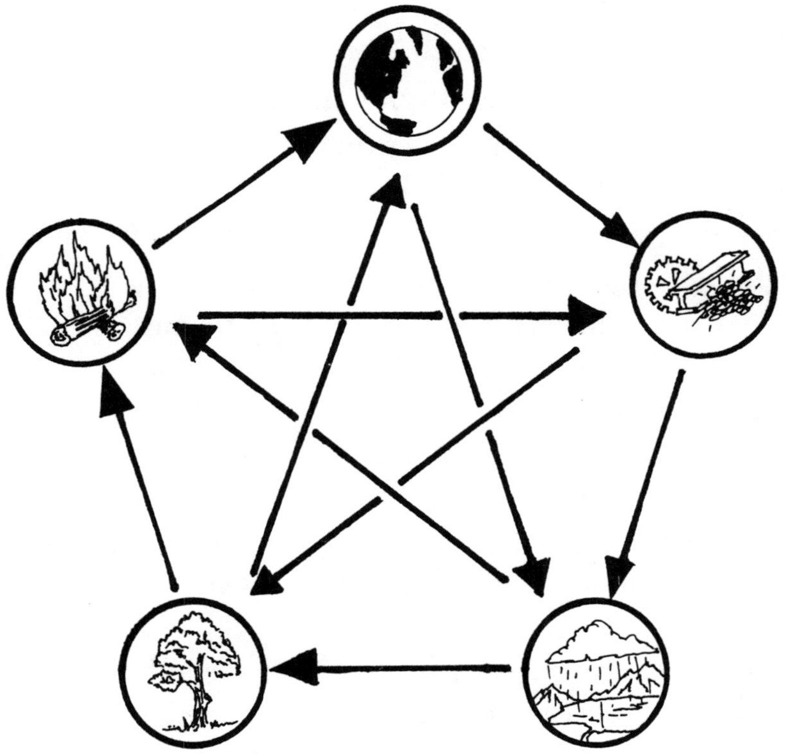

Shen and K'o Cycle: *This chart shows the K'o cycle in addition to the Shen cycle. The five-sided star shows the path of the K'o cycle. You can see from this chart that fire is the grandmother of metal according to the K'o cycle, and the mother of earth, according to the Shen cycle.*

Another way to understand the K'o cycle is to see the relationships between the elements in this way:

WOOD IS THE GRANDMOTHER OF EARTH
EARTH IS THE GRANDMOTHER OF WATER
WATER IS THE GRANDMOTHER OF FIRE
FIRE IS THE GRANDMOTHER OF METAL
METAL IS THE GRANDMOTHER OF WOOD

Just as I mentioned in discussing the Shen cycle, there are times when you may need to treat an element which precedes the element that you've chosen as needing the most attention. In the Shen cycle, that would be the mother. There may be times when you want to follow the path of the K'o cycle and tonify or strengthen the grandmother of the element you are working on. For example, if the element in which your primary issues arise is too strong, you may be able to sedate it by tonifying the grandmother. This would result in the grandmother increasing her control over the grandson and thus reducing the grandson's energy. If, instead, the element you're focusing on is lacking in energy, you may want to sting the son in addition to the element itself. You will note that the son is the grandmother of the grandmother, so that this treatment follows the K'o cycle—tonifying the great-great grandmother tempers the grandmother, thus allowing the original deficient element the freedom to increase.

Bee stings are a potent way to tonify or strengthen a pathway or point. Because bee stings are highly energizing, they cannot be used to sedate a point or a pathway; this is a technique which requires the skilled use of acupuncture needles. If you believe that sedating a pathway is an important approach, you may want to consider tonifying the grandmother as described above.

Excessive control can eventually bring about a condition called Aggressive Energy. This imbalance is considered one of the major blocks; these blocks and their treatments are discussed in Chapter 9. If you find yourself pulled between very high energy states and serious depression, this could be due to an imbalance in which excessive energy in one part of your system dampens energy in another. Such swings in mood or energy level might be treated by both addressing the K'o cycle and by draining Aggressive Energy. Some people's focus on a particular area—in which they may either excel or obsess—can cause other areas in their life to suffer. If the elements you choose in the following chapter have a grandmother-son relationship, then you may want to consider the K'o cycle as you choose the pathways to sting.

THE CAUSATIVE FACTOR
(TREATING THE CAUSE AND NOT THE SYMPTOMS)

In addition to all the blocks that can develop along the way on our own journey to wholeness, a trained traditional acupuncturist will be looking to see where each person was originally knocked off balance in childhood. This could have been something like pneumonia, a high fever, or even a death in the family. This original imbalance or illness is called the causative factor (CF). It is the first element that went out of balance and stayed out of balance. This will be the weak link in the chain, the one most likely to go under stress. The CF is where you can go to gain access to the person in treatment and everything else changes.

I need to emphasize here, that it is very difficult, or perhaps impossible, to diagnose a patient's CF from reading a book. A trained acupuncturist can make such a determination, and then only with a face to face consultation with the person. Such a diagnosis is based on a myriad of considerations, such as the color on the face, the sound of the voice, the smell of the body, and from a sense as to which emotion is most out of balance. The goal of this book is not to help you definitively arrive at the CF, but to help you see which element may be most out of balance for you. This gives you a good place to focus your treatment.

Imagine that each person is like a desert. Now think about this: what can I bring to this person that will make the biggest difference? If I bring plants (wood) to a desert, it will not change anything. If I bring more heat (fire) to a desert, it will not make a difference. If I bring more dirt (earth), to a desert nothing changes. If I bring metal (air) to the desert, it stays the same. But, if I bring water to the desert, it will change everything! And it's the same way with people. You need to decide which element will make the biggest difference to the person. It is usually the element that was the first one to be knocked off balance. Please keep in mind that it may not be the element that is "screaming" the loudest or has the most symptoms.

The decision as to which element is the primary one or the CF is totally based on the color, the sound, the odor and the emotion. That is why it is hard to diagnose yourself from a book. The CF is only truly diagnosed by a trained acupuncturist who is able to see the patient.

Understanding the balance of energy in the body, where distortions and blocks have become ingrained, and which are primary, helps you get to the root of the problem. You need to get to the root cause and not just treat on the surface. If you think of a person as a tree, you must treat the roots and not just the branches. If you nourish the roots the branches will become healthy again. If you just treat the branches you can't help the whole tree.

Traditional acupuncture aims to get to the root cause. The body is seen as a dynamic whole, a network of interacting energies. So, if you support the place where the person was originally knocked off balance, the body will heal itself and the symptoms will disappear on their own. As in the domino theory, if you tap the first domino, all the others fall on their own.

Let's take another example. Look at your car. If the oil light in your car is flashing, you wouldn't want the mechanic to cut the wire. Although it would prevent the light from flashing, you would rather the mechanic get down to the root cause, wouldn't you? Where your health is concerned, even more than for your car, you'd certainly want someone to be able to find the root cause of your condition and not just cover up the problem. Although it is tempting to go for the quick fix, I believe in my heart that we all truly want to be healed from the inside and not just on the surface.

Any illness invites us home to take a moment and sift through levels of our experience and be open to needed changes. When illness arises we must stop, look, and listen. When we experience dis-ease a message is trying to come through which we haven't received yet. This message will persist, increasing in intensity and frequency, until we see it. We can choose to be open to it, to avoid it, or even hate it. Any resistance can create a conflict or struggle and this will determine the degree of our illness. Remember, all sickness is homesickness. We are all Dorothys and Totos from "The Wizard of Oz." We are all just trying to find our way home again, home to ourselves.

THE CHINESE CLOCK

Every 24 hours the *Ch'i* flows through the whole body via the 12 main meridians. Each meridian is at its peak for two hours, and 12 hours later it will be at its lowest point. This is called the Law of Midday-Midnight or the Law of the Chinese Clock.

The theory behind the Chinese Clock can give you very valuable information for understanding yourself and others. If there is a weakness, excess, or block on one of the pathways, you may get symptoms at the same time every day. Patients may make comments like this:

> "I'm always tired in the late afternoon."
> "I am not a morning person."
> "I am a night person."

You can take advantage of this clock. By treating a pathway when it is at its peak, you can get a more powerful response. This can be increased even more by treating the meridian at the right time of day in the right season. This is called a horary treatment. A horary treatment is done by treating the home element point—the point on that pathway which is the same element as the pathway, i.e., a wood point on a wood pathway.

Let's say you want to strengthen the heart pathway. The time of day for the heart meridian is 11 a.m.—1 p.m. So you would have your patient come to see you at that time of day. And it's even better if they can come in at that time of day in the summer, because that is the season that goes with the heart. Since the heart is part of the fire element, you will want to treat the fire point on that pathway. That is what I meant when I said that you will treat the home element point on the pathway. If you were treating a wood pathway, you would be looking for the wood point on the wood pathway. Another name for a home element point is called a horary point. There is only one horary point on each pathway.

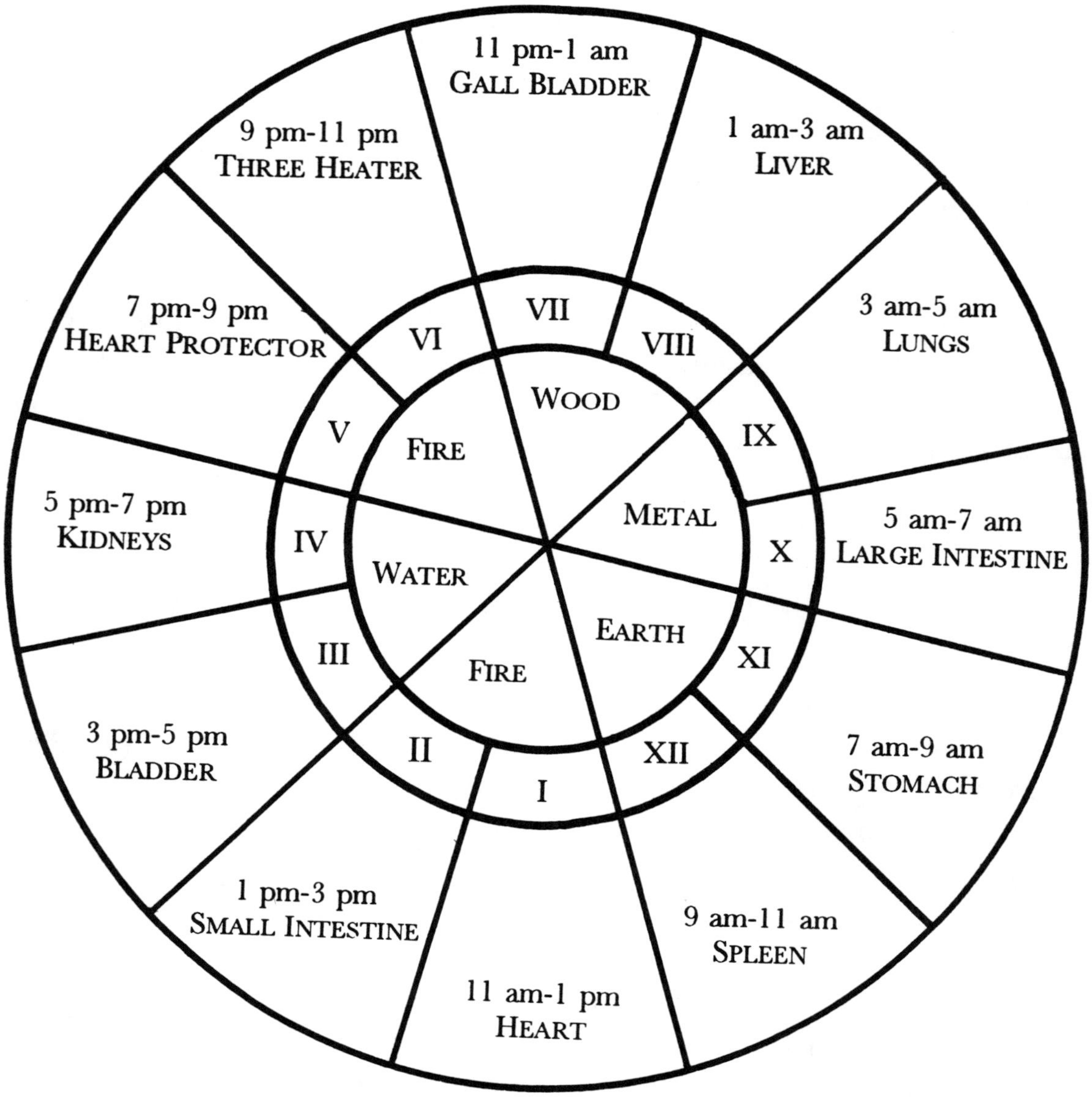

The Chinese Clock: *Because the energy moves through all twelve meridians in a 24-hour day, each pathway is at its peak for two hours. If a particular pathway is deficient, you may feel better during the time of day of that pathway. If a pathway has excess energy, then your symptoms may intensify during that time of day. For example, someone with deficient energy in the heart may feel better around lunch time. Someone with excess energy in the liver may be unable to sleep between 1 a.m. and 3 a.m. The times on this chart refer to "sun-time." During daylight savings time, be sure to subtract an hour.*

CHAPTER 6

FINDING YOURSELF WITHIN THE FIVE ELEMENTS

Please circle or underline any symptoms listed on the next two pages that relate to you. When you are all done, you will be ready to select which one of the five elements (Wood, Fire, Earth, Metal, or Water) seems the most out of balance for you. Consider the seriousness of the symptoms selected in each element as well as the number. This will suggest the element that you turn to first. At this point you will turn to the section that goes with that element. For example, if you have chosen to work with the Wood element first, then turn to the section of this chapter entitled Wood. You will then continue to underline the characteristics that relate to you.

Some diseases are thought to primarily manifest themselves in a particular element. The Chinese believe, for example, that MS, arthritis, and other chronic diseases can often be treated on the earth . . . spleen and stomach, and the wood . . . gall bladder and liver pathways. Each element is affected by a particular climate; the earth is affected by dampness, the wood, affected by wind. The Chinese believe that dampness and wind have invaded the body to produce what they consider to be rheumatoid conditions—MS, arthritis, and other similar chronic diseases. It is important, though, to learn to understand each individual person. As Hippocrates said, it's more important to treat the person with the disease than the disease. Only in this way can you get to the underlying cause and treat the whole picture.

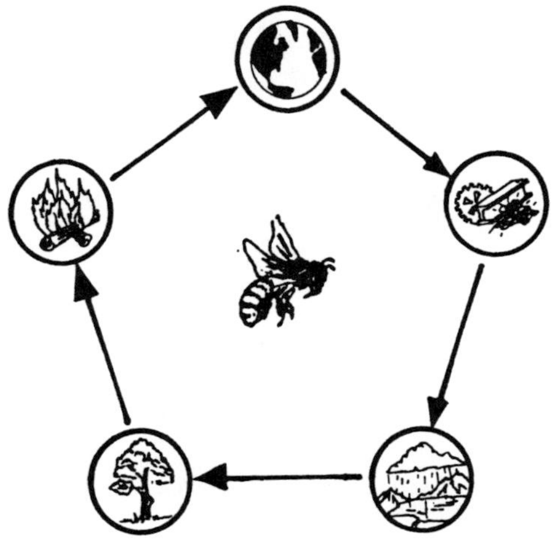

Circle each symptom you experience listed for each of the five elements—

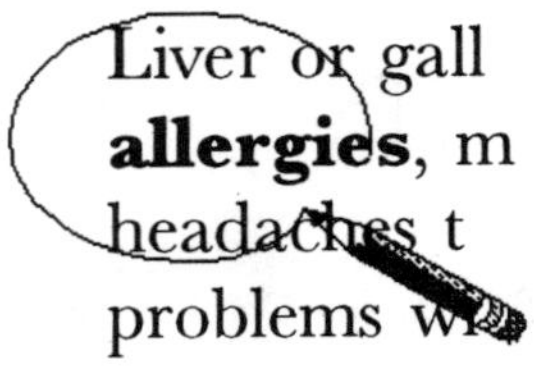

—then determine which element you appear to be having the most trouble with based on the number and severity of the conditions circled. Then turn to the section for that element.

POTENTIAL MANIFESTATIONS OF IMBALANCES IN THE FIVE ELEMENTS:

WOOD

Liver or gall bladder problems, hepatitis, jaundice, allergies, migraines, headaches (either one-sided or headaches that feel like a tight band around the head); problems with tendons and ligaments, lack of coordination, MS, fibromyalgia; migrating pains (pains that move around), dry or brittle nails/nail biting, chronic fatigue syndrome or Epstein-Barre; eye problems; anger, irritability, impatience, frustration, needing a sense of direction, trouble making decisions, procrastination, addictions; a creative person, artists, singers, dancers, writers; likes or dislikes spring, green, sour taste; may be a night person or may wake up or have trouble sleeping between 11 p.m. and 3 a.m.

FIRE

High fevers (especially in childhood, i.e., rheumatic fever, scarlet fever, measles), issues with hot and cold; heart problems, circulatory problems; small intestine problems; sexual problems or sexual abuse; fibromyalgia; stuttering, feelings of chaos and panic, issues of control (fear of being around a controlling person, needing to be in control, feeling out of control), feeling "spacey" or confused, can't sort things out, has too many options and doesn't know what to do, "absent-minded professor," issues of trust, fear of being hurt/rejected, feeling unloved, relationship issues, wanting unconditional love, feeling responsible for everyone else (like the conductor of an orchestra, "if I'm not taking care of things, everything falls apart"); likes or dislikes summer, red, bitter tastes, may use humor a lot or laugh a lot, "class clown," "comedian," or a lack of laughter and joy; trouble falling asleep; issues between 11 a.m. and 3p.m. and 7 p.m. and 11 p.m.

EARTH

Stomach and spleen problems, digestive troubles, vomiting, nausea, belching, burping, hiatal hernias, ulcers, anorexia/bulimia; lumps, cysts, (especially breast); spinning and dizziness, craving sweets, diabetes or low blood sugar, pancreas problems; leg cramps, muscle problems, MS, feeling very tired and heavy, (like a slug—just can't move, "I just can't get out of this chair . . . I can't even lift my arm"), chronic fatigue syndrome; overweight or unusual distribution of weight; obsessions, "poor me," never satisfied, not feeling centered or grounded, nightmares, smothering someone else or fear of being smothered emotionally, feeling needy, wanting sympathy, needing to be understood or feeling misunderstood, a caretaker or wanting to be taken care of, issues around mothering, nurturing and your relationship with your own mother; likes or dislikes the color yellow, sweets, humidity, "a morning person" or dislikes the morning; issues between 7 a.m. and 11 a.m.

METAL

Lung problems (especially in childhood), bronchitis, pneumonia, pleurisy, asthma, allergies, coughs, sore throats, mononucleosis, environmental illness; large intestine problems, diarrhea, spastic colon, constipation, hernia, excess mucus, skin problems; difficulties with the nose or sense of smell, sinus problems, headaches; feeling cut-off and alone, fear of being alone and a need for connections, or a loner, low self-esteem and self-worth, wears excess metal jewelry; likes vacations to the mountains, helped by meditation, tends to focus on the negative, complains a lot, the wailing wall syndrome, living in the past, sadness and unresolved grief and loss (divorces, deaths, moving to a new area—the loss of friends or support system), perfectionism, judgmental and unforgiving, has trouble letting go, can never throw anything out or likes to keep things very clean; likes or dislikes autumn, white, spicy foods, dryness; may wake up between 3 a.m. and 7 a.m., or have dreams of sharp objects, flying, death and dying.

WATER

Bladder and kidney problems, spine problems, spinal meningitis, brain problems, epilepsy; combination of low back and knee problems, blood pressure issues, teeth problems, excess perspiration, ear disorders; environmental illness; feeling burnt out, wants a vacation (especially to the water); fear, anxiety, panic attacks, fear of bridges, darkness, claustrophobia, lack of fear, feeling overwhelmed, no ambition/will; afraid of bees, spiders and other insects; likes or dislikes winter, the cold, salty foods, the color blue or black, issues between 3 p.m. and 7 p.m.

WOOD

You have chosen to work on the wood element. The wood element has two pathways associated with it, the gall bladder and the liver. This section is designed to give you the information you need to decide if one of those pathways is more important for you than the other.

Please circle or underline any characteristics or symptoms that relate to you on the gall bladder pathway and then on the liver pathway. When you are done, select the pathway you want to begin with. Turn to the treatment plan for that pathway and follow the directions. When you are ready, you can switch to the other pathway.

If you cannot decide which pathway you want to start with, it is OK to work on both pathways simultaneously. Remember to keep good, clear records of what you do. That way, if you have good results you can duplicate your experience. Also, good records will enable us to gather more information to help others in the future.

After you have worked on the wood element for awhile, you may want to consider starting on another element. You can always come back to the wood pathways when you need to.

You may want to pay extra special attention to the wood element in the season associated with it, spring, and also when you notice symptoms that go with the wood element.

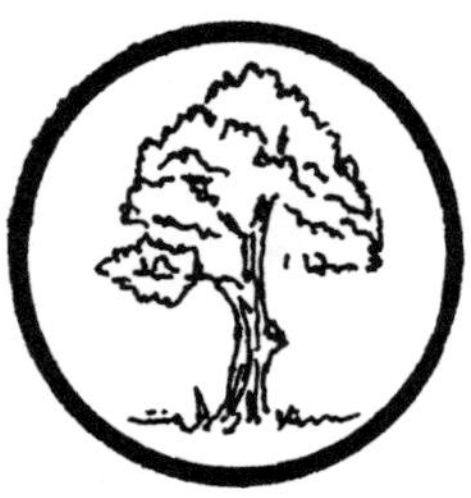

"LET'S FACE IT, THE DOCTOR'S KNOW NOTHING ABOUT MS; WE LIVE WITH IT!"

Judy's Story

When I first started taking the bee stings, I was not expecting any results. "It's not going to do any good, but I've got nothing to lose!" I was very skeptical. I was intentionally negative to avoid the placebo effect. I was willing to do it for six months. "Let's see what happens," I thought to myself. My expectations were low on purpose. I didn't want to get my hopes up.

I developed the "healing crisis" after the first few sessions and had flu-like symptoms for a day and a half. Within the first two months, I noticed my energy had increased. Gradually I noticed that my stamina was much better. I could stand for a longer period of time. The most important improvement came in the fourth month. I started to regain control of my bladder. For the first time in several years, I was able to sleep through the night without getting up to urinate!

One day I was feeling angry and I asked Amber if there were any sting locations for anger. She said yes and promptly stung me on the liver pathway. And believe it or not, those stings really made a difference!

I'm glad that I met Amber. I know I am part of a healing community whenever I visit her home. Bee stings are certainly worth a try.

Judy is a librarian. She has written a children's book called, "My Mom is NOT Weird!," to be published by Crystal River Press in the winter of 1994-5. It is about a mother who has MS and goes to talk to her child's class at school. A.R.

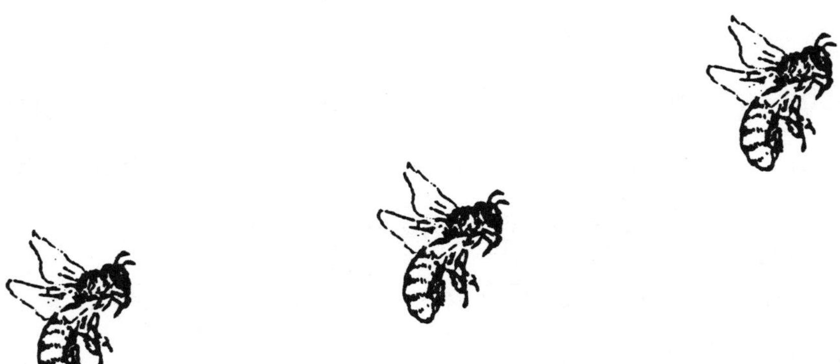

THE GALL BLADDER

Circle or underline any item(s) on this page that you feel relate to you:

POSITIVE QUALITIES:

When the pathway is in balance, the person makes good decisions; has good judgment, good vision, good sense of direction; concerned with fairness and justice; ability to assert self; flexible; good coordination; good organizational skills; wants to grow, able to move forward and see clearly; may be very creative, such as artists, dancers, or musicians.

PHYSICAL CONDITIONS (ESPECIALLY IN CHILDHOOD) THAT MAY CAUSE OR SIGNAL AN IMBALANCE IN THE GALLBLADDER:

When this pathway is out of balance, the person may have these physical problems: issues with the gall bladder; eye problems; problems of ligaments and tendons; i.e., MS, myofacial pain, fibromyalgia, bursitis, arthritis, frozen joints (shoulders, elbows, knees or especially hip); coordination problems; one-sided complaints (especially one-sided headaches), pains that migrate and move around; alcohol or drug-related problems; low energy; many scars (especially large scars—any time there is a scar, the gall bladder has to make a decision on how to heal the person—how soon someone gets well from any illness or injury depends on the gall bladder); dry or brittle nails, nail biting; allergies; addictions; headaches due to anger; buzzing in the ears; migrating pains; dry, brittle nails; nail biting; difficulty with any symptoms or issues between 11 p.m. and 3 a.m. (waking up or being more creative in those hours); likes or dislikes wind, spring, sour foods, the color green. The person shouts alot or has a very quiet voice that sounds "breathy."

EMOTIONAL/SPIRITUAL IMBALANCES OF THE GALLBLADDER:

When this pathway is out of balance the person may have the following emotional/spiritual problems: difficulty making decisions; confusion or "wishy-washiness"; can't finish projects; easily intimidated, non-assertive, shy, weak, procrastination, lack of direction, no growth (artists who feel blocked and can't grow, "writers' block"); frustration, anger, impatience; very judgmental, rigid, punishing and judging others; sergeant type of a person with inconstancy, "hard on the outside and soft on the inside"; pushy; negative; no "give"; blind to reality around him/her; very in tune to fairness—go crazy if things are not fair; has trouble with hierarchy; agitation, "can't sit still," fighting in school, rebellious in childhood, can't stand anything out of order; splits—left/right, top/bottom—feels pulled apart, identity issues; pays either a great deal of attention to details or no attention at all; difficulty with timing or feeling that there is not enough time; career issues; soft voice but angry inside; screams a lot; depression—due to anger held in or frustration at lack of growth.

TO TREAT THE GALL BLADDER PATHWAY
➥ TURN TO PAGE 103

THE LIVER

Circle or underline any item(s) on this page that you feel relate to you:

POSITIVE QUALITIES:

When this pathway is in balance, the person excels in planning and organization, plans every activity for survival; guards the body from outside insults and inside toxicities; plans for the future (visual clarity and order); the architect who sees the big picture and makes plans and blueprints, and has goals; a person who has direction, knows where he's going and knows his place in life; sense of serenity, feels hopeful, wants to grow, able to break habits, can move forward, has hindsight, foresight, and insight; can put things in perspective; plans for growth and birth; stands tall against the wind, well-rooted; very hopeful; good muscle power to push through things.

PHYSICAL CONDITIONS (ESPECIALLY IN CHILDHOOD) THAT MAY CAUSE OR SIGNAL AN IMBALANCE IN THE LIVER :

When this pathway is out of balance, the person may have these physical problems: liver problems, hepatitis, jaundice, allergies, migraine headaches or headaches that feel like a tight band around the head; headaches when anger is stuck in the head; addictions to drugs or alcohol; problems with the immune system; problems with tendons and ligaments; MS, fibromyalgia, joint problems, rheumatic pains, pains that move around; eye problems (especially blurred vision); gynecological problems with blood flow; inability to recuperate, trouble bouncing back from illness; trouble getting up and sitting down; issues of glycolysis; problems with nails/nail biting; fatigue, achy limbs, difficulty with the wind; symptoms or issues between 1 a.m. and 3 a.m. (especially when waking then, or more creative then); likes or dislikes spring, sour food, the color green, and the wind. The person shouts alot or has a very quiet, "breathy" voice.

EMOTIONAL/SPIRITUAL IMBALANCES OF THE LIVER:

When this pathway is out of balance the person may have the following emotional/spiritual problems: trouble making plans, trouble when plans change, no clear goals, "has no future," deep sense of hopelessness, or jumping into the future, not living in the present; easily blown over, not rooted, trouble breaking habits, impatient, frustrated; over-planning, checks and rechecks to see if alarm is set, if stove is off, if door is locked; green with envy, very competitive, makes comparisons between self and others (comparing one's inside to someone else's outside), walking around aimlessly and "feeling lost"; people who have never really grown up, stuck in anger, really intense; career issues (has many different careers or "doesn't know what they want to be when they grow up"); very soft voice but angry inside, or screams a lot; angry at self (may cause auto-immune diseases), self-criticism; not being able to see the forest for the trees, losing sight of your goals, operating in the dark, can't see where you are going and therefore you are in the dark, easily irritated, angry, "don't bother me"; lack of focus, sitting on anger, sour grapes, sourpuss, relationships "go sour," addictive personality, depression when you can't see a future, holding anger in or feeling like you're not growing.

TO TREAT THE LIVER PATHWAY
➥ TURN TO PAGE 108

FIRE

You have chosen to work on the fire element. The fire element has four pathways associated with it: the heart, the small intestine, the heart protector, and the three heater. This section is designed to give you the information you need to decide if one of those pathways is more important for you than the others.

Please circle or underline any characteristics or symptoms that relate to you on each of the four pathways. When you are done, select the pathway you want to begin with. Turn to the treatment plan for that pathway and follow the directions.

When you are ready, you can begin to work on the other pathways. If you cannot decide which pathway you want to start with, it is OK to work on all of them simultaneously. But you must remember to keep good, clear records of what you do. That way, if you have good results you can duplicate your experience. Also, good records will enable us to gather more information to help others in the future.

After you have worked on the fire element for a while, you may want to choose another element to start on. You can always come back to the fire element when you need to.

You may want to pay extra special attention to the fire element during the season that is associated with it, summer, and when you are having symptoms that are related to it.

"I AM NO LONGER COLD!"

JEAN'S STORY

I was diagnosed as having MS in 1980, but probably had the disease for some years before that. I have been confined to a wheelchair since 1985. When my MS was diagnosed, my neurologist said that if I remained stable for three years, the disease probably wouldn't progress—become worse. But about three years later, my condition did start to deteriorate, and kept doing so, slowly. I have never taken any medicine for the MS, none being prescribed.

However, the deterioration has stopped in the past year, and I see signs of improvement in my physical condition. This seems clearly to be the result of bee sting therapy, aided by some acupuncture treatment. I have been getting bee stings since May 17, 1993, or a little over a year now. I get approximately 16-20 stings each time. At first it was three times a week and now it's twice a week. The stinging was started by Pat Wagner in Waldorf, MD. In the fall of 1993, I started going to Amber Rose in nearby Bethesda. I have been stung more than 2200 times to date.

I have seen definite improvement in my physical condition since these ministrations began. While my MS still keeps me in a wheelchair, there have been positive changes.

1. With my husband's help for balance, I can stand for up to two minutes. Before Bee Venom Therapy I would start to collapse almost as soon as I was aided to the standing position. Also, I can now pull myself to standing, fairly frequently, holding onto a firm vertical support. I couldn't do that before.

2. My right hand was tightly clenched and immovable before BVT. It is now mostly open all the time, and can be opened and closed by me or others with relative ease.

3. My legs can move apart fairly easily. Before, they were rigidly pushed together.

A short time after I started the bee stings with Amber, she began acupuncture treatments on me. Then I noticed I was no longer cold, which had been the case since I was 10 years old. That was when I had "two-three week measles" for the second time. For over 50 years, I have used a hot water bottle at night, and have nearly always worn a sweater, except during the hottest part of the day. After acupuncture and bee stings, I have now been warm for several months—across my upper back and shoulder blades, upper arms, and my legs and feet.

I am grateful for these gains. Bee stings and acupuncture work well together.

I'M VERY EXCITED BY THE PROGRESS JEAN HAS MADE! A.R.

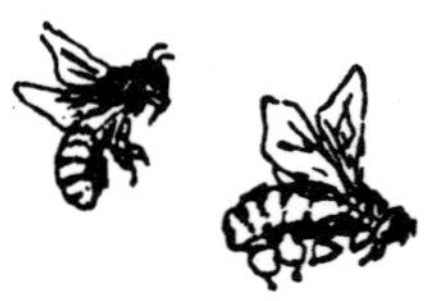

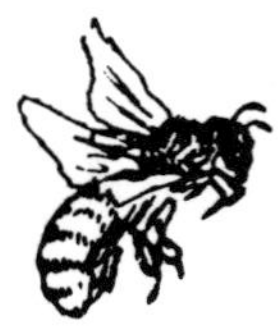

"I CAN OPEN MY HAND NOW FOR THE FIRST TIME IN 8 YEARS . . ."

THE HEART: THE SUPREME CONTROLLER

Circle or underline any item(s) on this page that you feel relate to you:

POSITIVE QUALITIES:

When this pathway is in balance, the person has integrity; is very responsible for coordinating the whole, like the conductor of an orchestra; treats each person as important; has a quality of selflessness and unconditional love; is very insightful and wise; has a need to communicate, care and give.

PHYSICAL CONDITIONS (ESPECIALLY IN CHILDHOOD) THAT MAY CAUSE OR SIGNAL AN IMBALANCE IN THE HEART:

When this pathway is out of balance, the person may have these physical problems: high fevers, especially scarlet fever, rheumatic fever, measles; heart murmurs and congenital heart and circulation problems; a history of electric shock treatments, electrical accidents, shocks, being struck by lightning; pain down the arm and up the throat; a history of sexual abuse, fibromyalgia, being in a fire; feeling better or worse between 11 a.m. and 1 p.m.; likes or dislikes the bitter taste, fires, the color red, summer, and heat. The sound of the voice is either happy (with lots of laughter) or is flat (lack of laugh).

EMOTIONAL/SPIRITUAL IMBALANCES OF THE HEART:

When this pathway is out of balance, the person may have the following emotional/spiritual problems: wants to be the center of attention; feels overwhelmed with too much responsibility; may treat a person like a thing; likes to be in control or has an issue with control, may feel out of control (a feeling of panic); defensive, may experience themselves as a failure, feels betrayed; coldness on every level, (physical, emotional, or spiritual); keeps busy; denial of the whole, lack of joy: "I feel dead or empty"; everything looks OK on the outside, but everything is mechanical on the inside; "I feel like my heart is encased in cement," "I feel drained of life"; if this pathway is out of balance, you may get symptoms associated with the other elements and other pathways—if you see yourself in all of the elements, and can't decide which element is your primary issue, it may be the heart.

TO TREAT THE HEART PATHWAY
➥ TURN TO PAGE 111

THE SMALL INTESTINES

Circle or underline any item(s) on this page that you feel relate to you:

POSITIVE QUALITIES:

When this pathway is in balance, the person is concerned with separating the pure from the impure, sends the pure food to the spleen for distribution and the garbage to the colon for elimination; ability to sort out all of life's experiences; ability to transform suffering into joy (an alchemist); to see clearly, to know the difference between self and others, knows what belongs where, "knows what's best and what's destructive to me."

PHYSICAL CONDITIONS (ESPECIALLY IN CHILDHOOD) THAT MAY CAUSE OR SIGNAL AN IMBALANCE IN THE SMALL INTESTINE :

When this pathway is out of balance, the person may have these physical problems: high fevers, measles; fibromyalgia; ear problems; small intestine blockage, digestive problems, or boils; being in a fire; feels better or worse between 1:00 p.m. and 3:00 p.m.; likes or dislikes the color red, heat, summer, and the bitter taste. The person's voice will have alot of laughter in it or may be flat with no joy at all.

EMOTIONAL/SPIRITUAL IMBALANCES OF THE SMALL INTESTINE:

When this pathway is out of balance, the person may have the following emotional/spiritual problems: feeling "spacey" or confused, can't sort things out, life is cluttered (like an old Victorian house), too many options and the person doesn't know what to do, "maybe I'll do this, no . . . maybe I'll do that . . . no, I think I'll do that"; absent-minded professor; wanting to run away from problems when they don't know what to do; joyless, feeling polluted, feeling their energy is clogged up; problems of separation, sorting and choosing poorly, (leaving you in situations or relationships where you may get hurt or stay with people who are not good for you.)

TO TREAT THE SMALL INTESTINE PATHWAY
➥ TURN TO PAGE 114

THE HEART PROTECTOR

Circle or underline any item(s) on this page that you feel relate to you:

POSITIVE QUALITIES:

When this pathway is in balance, the heart is well protected from the bumps and bruises of life, the person doesn't her get feelings hurt easily (there is good protection); he carries the essence of the heart out to others; good sexual function; good circulatory function; the "gatekeeper of the castle moat," knows when to open and close the drawbridge and let people in and out, knows how to be intimate, doesn't feel vulnerable—feels well protected.

PHYSICAL CONDITIONS (ESPECIALLY IN CHILDHOOD) THAT MAY CAUSE OR SIGNAL AN IMBALANCE IN THE HEART PROTECTOR :

When this pathway is out of balance, the person may have the following physical conditions: high fevers, especially rheumatic fever, scarlet fever, measles; heart problems, sexual problems, sexual abuse, rapes; fibromyalgia; shoulders tend to slump forward; circulation problems, interruption in cardiac rhythm, angina, palpitations, cold hands and cold feet; problems between 7:00 p.m. and 9:00 p.m.; likes or dislikes the color red, summer, heat, fires, and the bitter taste. The person's voice is either happy and filled with laughter or flat (lack of joy).

EMOTIONAL/SPIRITUAL IMBALANCES OF THE HEART PROTECTOR:

When this pathway is out of balance, the person may experience the following emotional/spiritual problems: issues of trust, fear of being hurt/rejected, feeling unloved, relationship issues, wanting unconditional love, feeling unprotected and vulnerable, easily hurt, wearing your heart on your shirtsleeve, not feeling safe, loss of memory to protect oneself, lack of intimacy or craving intimacy, putting walls up to protect oneself, self-deception to protect oneself, issues of chemistry in a relationship, heartbreak in a relationship, sexual issues (impotence, frigidity); fear of being cold; depression due to feeling unloved or that you've displeased someone.

TO TREAT THE HEART PROTECTOR PATHWAY
➥ TURN TO PAGE 118

THE "THREE HEATER"

Circle or underline any item(s) on this page that you feel relate to you:

POSITIVE QUALITIES:

When this pathway is in balance, the person may be good at balance and harmony, enjoys being the peacemaker; works to create a perfect environment, a networker, good at receiving and transmitting information (a TV or radio announcer), good conversationalist, good debater; perfect hostess, loves to touch/hug and be touched/hugged, enjoys groups, keeps the family in touch, sends birthday cards etc., brings warmth to situations.

PHYSICAL CONDITIONS (ESPECIALLY IN CHILDHOOD) THAT MAY CAUSE OR SIGNAL AN IMBALANCE IN THE THREE HEATER:

When this pathway is out of balance, the person may experience the following physical problems: high fevers, measles, feeling too hot or too cold (the thermostat within the body is out of balance), cold hands and cold feet; fibromyalgia; affected by the environment (a butcher going in and out of the freezer; a person going in and out of a hot tub, sauna, using an electric blanket, etc.); feels hot and cold, has fear of cold and wears many layers of clothing or feels warm and wears less clothing then most people on a cold day, breathing problems due to not enough heat in the lungs; withdraws heat, warmth from organs (like pelvis—difficulty conceiving); being in a fire, speech impediments or stuttering, hearing problems, problems between 9 p.m. and 11 p.m.; likes or dislikes bitter taste, the color red, summer, and heat. The person has a joyful and laughing voice or one that is flat with no joy.

EMOTIONAL/SPIRITUAL IMBALANCES OF THE THREE HEATER:

When this pathway is out of balance, the person may experience the following emotional/spiritual problems: having to be the peacemaker in your family and not liking it; not feeling loved ("I have all these friends—but I don't feel loved"), constantly trying to connect to be loved, inability to make social contacts, can't discriminate between social and intimate contacts, feeling that you're nice to them one day and they think you are their best friend), or they can't reach out ("I don't know anybody"), they always have some excuse for not reaching out or they hide in their one relationship and have trouble reaching out from it; withdrawing love from others, depression due to feeling unloved or that you've displeased someone; pulling back one's love or needing to give out a lot of warmth and love; may have difficulty with groups or public speaking, stuttering, speech impediments.

TO TREAT THE THREE HEATER PATHWAY
➥ TURN TO PAGE 121

EARTH

You have chosen to work on the earth element. The earth element has two pathways associated with it, the stomach and the spleen. This section is designed to give you the information you need to decide if one of those pathways is more important for you than the other.

Please circle or underline any characteristics or symptoms that relate to you on the stomach pathway and then on the spleen pathway. When you are done, select the pathway you want to begin with. Turn to the treatment plan for that pathway and follow the directions. When you are ready, you can work on the other pathway.

If you cannot decide which pathway you want to start with, it is OK to work on both pathways simultaneously. Remember to keep good, clear records of what you do. That way, if you have good results you can duplicate your experience. Also, good records will enable us to gather more information to help others in the future.

After you have worked on the earth element for a while, you may want to choose another element to work on. You can always come back to the earth element whenever you need to .

You may want to pay extra special attention to the earth element in the season associated with it, late summer, or when you are having symptoms related to the earth element.

"I LOVE MY BEE STINGS!"

MEG'S STORY

As I lay on the acupuncture table waiting for Amber to sting me not just with needles but with live bees, I thought to myself, "Boy, Meg, this is probably the most unusual thing you've ever done." How would people react if I told them, "Oh, by the way, I get stung once a week by bees (on purpose?)" But when Amber—a gifted and natural healer, whom I trusted implicitly—told me what she was doing with bee stings, I said, "Sign me up!" So, once a week, I travel to Bethesda to get my needles and my stingers.

Initially, the swelling and itching were bothersome, but after a month of weekly stings, they don't bother me at all. In fact, I love my bee stings! I experience an incredible feeling of well being and happiness after each session. I also have much more energy. I suffer from endometriosis, and the regular stingings have greatly improved the chronic pain I have. Each month it gets better and better. In addition, Amber has been stinging me on my appendectomy scar and it's disappearing. These bees are somethin' else!

I HAVE KNOWN MEG FOR MANY YEARS. SHE'S A KIND AND GENTLE PERSON WHO GOES THE EXTRA MILE FOR OTHERS. I'M SO GLAD THAT THE BEES ARE MAKING A DIFFERENCE IN HER LIFE. SHE DESERVES THE BEST! A.R.

THE STOMACH

Circle or underline any item(s) on this page that you feel relate to you:

POSITIVE QUALITIES:

When this pathway is in balance, the person has a good digestive system, receives and provides nourishment to the body; is very nurturing and empathetic; integrates and processes well; reliable, steady, centered.

PHYSICAL CONDITIONS (ESPECIALLY IN CHILDHOOD) THAT MAY CAUSE OR SIGNAL AN IMBALANCE IN THE STOMACH:

When this pathway is out of balance, the person may experience the following physical problems: digestion problems, belching, burping, anorexia, bulimia, cramps, leg pains, muscle problems, MS, chronic fatigue syndrome; nausea, vomiting; diabetes, hypoglycemia, headaches due to hypoglycemia; loves sweets, needing to chewing gum or have something sweet in one's mouth; overweight, unusual distribution of weight, lumps, difficult pregnancies, miscarriages; hiatal hernia; problems between 7:00 a.m.—9:00 a.m., "a morning person" or "definitely not a morning person"; likes or dislikes humidity, late summer, and the colors yellow, orange and brown. The sound of the voice has either a singing quality to it or it is monotone.

EMOTIONAL/SPIRITUAL IMBALANCES OF THE STOMACH:

When this pathway is out of balance, the person may experience the following emotional/spiritual problems: craving sympathy, empathy, very needy and clingy, or taking care of everyone else but not asking for help yourself; lack of centeredness, never feeling satisfied, "poor me," craving to be understood or feeling misunderstood, "hungry or starved" for love or sex (pawing), caretaker, needing to be needed, depression due to feeling needy and starving, and having trouble with "the empty nest syndrome."

TO TREAT THE STOMACH PATHWAY
➥ TURN TO PAGE 126

THE SPLEEN

Circle or underline any item(s) on this page that you feel relate to you:

POSITIVE QUALITIES:

When this pathway is in balance, the person has good energy, maintains good blood sugar levels, lymphatic system in good shape, the body has the ability to protect itself; a sense of fulfillment with life, enjoys bringing children into the world.

PHYSICAL CONDITIONS (ESPECIALLY IN CHILDHOOD) THAT MAY CAUSE OR SIGNAL AN IMBALANCE IN THE SPLEEN:

When this pathway is out of balance, the person may experience the following physical problems: muscle problems, MS, feeling sluggish, chronic tiredness, chronic fatigue syndrome, listlessness, feels unable to pick up their hand, "my legs can't carry me where I want to go," heaviness, spinning, dizziness, craves or dislikes sweets, diabetes, hypoglycemia and blood sugar issues, including headaches; long term chronic illness that doesn't seem to have much cause; overweight and unusual distribution of weight, leg pain, a sagging feeling; trouble at 9 a.m.—11 a.m. or loves 9 a.m.—11 a.m.; likes or dislikes humidity, late summer, and the colors yellow, orange and brown. The person's voice is either singing or monotone.

EMOTIONAL/SPIRITUAL IMBALANCES OF THE SPLEEN:

When this pathway is out of balance, the person may experience the following emotional/spiritual problems: inability to cope with little daily things, inability to stop obsessiveness, belaboring issues, paying attention to petty details;

nightmares, especially with aspect of things spinning (going in circles); not carrying things to fruition, can't carry fetus to full term; giving too much, not taking care of oneself, smothering, overly sweet; paying too much attention to the body, lots of symptoms and no one can find a cause; very needy, almost draining, holding onto one's children, lack of peacefulness, depression due to fatigue or feeling needy (starving, tired).

TO TREAT THE SPLEEN PATHWAY
➥ TURN TO PAGE 133

METAL

You have chosen to work on the metal element. The metal element has two pathways associated with it, the lung and the colon. This section is designed to give you the information you need to decide if one of those pathways is more important for you than the other.

Please circle or underline any characteristics or symptoms that relate to you on the lung pathway and then on the colon pathway. When you are done, select the pathway you want to begin with. Turn to the treatment plan for that pathway and follow the directions. When you are ready, you can start on the other pathway.

If you cannot decide which pathway you want to start with, it is OK to work on both pathways simultaneously. Remember to keep good, clear records of what you do. That way, if you have good results you can duplicate your experience. Also, good records will enable us to gather more information to help others in the future.

After you have worked on this element for a while you might want to consider choosing another element to start on. You can always come back to the metal element when you need to.

You may want to pay extra special attention to the metal element in the season associated with it, the autumn, or when you are having symptoms related to the metal element.

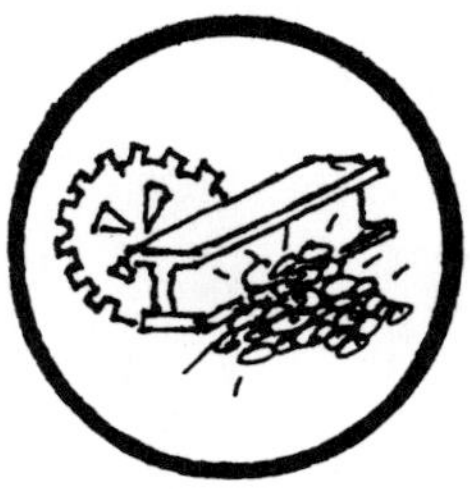

"I RODE MY BICYCLE 17 MILES WITHOUT WHEEZING!"

KEELY'S STORY

I have had Asthma since I was a child. I have taken a great deal of medicine over the years. A friend of mine told me about Amber. I decided to try some acupuncture with her. It really helped my breathing. One day I mentioned to her that I was having a problem with eczema. She suggested I take some royal jelly internally. I got some at the health food store and I was amazed that my skin condition disappeared.

Every time I went to Amber's house I was always curious about the bees. I was fascinated by her indoor observation hive. We talked about trying to get some bee venom as an inhalant for my Asthma, but were unable to find a good source of this. One day I decided I wanted to experience the bee stings. I was very impressed with the results. My breathing has been much easier. I need a lot less medicine these days. I hope some day to be off it completely. Just the other day I was able to ride my bicycle for 17 miles without wheezing. I'm all for the bees!

KEELY IS A VERY ENERGETIC YOUNG WOMAN WHO HAS A LOVE FOR LIFE AND A HEART OF JOY. HER EXCITEMENT ABOUT WHAT I'M DOING IS CONTAGIOUS. A.R.

THE LUNGS

Circle or underline any item(s) on this page that you feel relate to you:

POSITIVE QUALITIES:

When this pathway is in balance, the person feels very connected to the universe and to God, really into quality, brilliance, self-worth; easily inspired and gives inspiration to others; ability to receive and welcome; good relations with father; a sense of rhythmic order of life, aware of what is precious in life; "he is my rock of Gibraltar," rock-like structure, steadiness; good with finances; able to give and receive; never feels alone.

PHYSICAL CONDITIONS (ESPECIALLY IN CHILDHOOD) THAT MAY CAUSE OR SIGNAL AN IMBALANCE IN THE LUNGS:

When this pathway is out of balance, the person may experience the following physical problems: lung problems, pleurisy, pneumonia, bronchitis, asthma, allergies, skin problems (the skin is the third lung), coughs, sore throats, mononucleosis; leukemia, environmental illness; excess mucus, dairy allergies, craving spicy foods or has trouble with it; smokers; congestion headaches; trouble sleeping between 3 a.m. and 5 a.m.; likes or dislikes dryness, the color white, and autumn; wears alot of metal jewelry or can't wear any. The sound of the person's voice is sad and weepy.

EMOTIONAL/SPIRITUAL IMBALANCES OF THE LUNG:

When this pathway is out of balance, the person may experience the following emotional/spiritual problems: difficulty receiving love and compliments, feeling cut off, a loner, lack of self-worth, feeling inadequate; difficult relationship with guru, looking for what his own father never gave him, looking to fill emptiness or a void, lonely, wanting to be special, feeling unappreciated, feeling unworthy, guilty; trouble with money issues; negativity, depression, "going manic," soaring to the heights and plunging to the depths; helped by meditation; smokers who feel as if their cigarettes are like a companion ("maybe now that I'm in this relationship I'll be able to give up smoking"), grief, loss, sadness, the pain of giving someone something and they don't or can't receive it; likes vacations in the mountains; fear of being alone; speech difficulties, a weak voice or trouble getting the words out, or a "know-it-all" who feels much superior to everyone else; wears excess jewelry.

TO TREAT THE LUNG PATHWAY
➡ TURN TO PAGE 137

THE COLON (LARGE INTESTINE)

Circle or underline any item(s) on this page that you feel relate to you:

POSITIVE QUALITIES:

When this pathway is in balance, the person lets go easily and without effort, faith that quality and abundance are available, able to detach when necessary; able to grieve and then let go; feels special and unique; large intestine moves well; neat and clean; loves the mountains, feels connected to the universe, goes for quality; knows what to retain and what to let go.

PHYSICAL CONDITIONS (ESPECIALLY IN CHILDHOOD) THAT MAY CAUSE OR SIGNAL AN IMBALANCE IN THE COLON:

When this pathway is out of balance, the person may experience the following physical problems: severe diarrhea or constipation, dysentery, spastic colon; hernias; mononucleosis; leukemia, environmental illness; excess mucus, dairy allergies, difficulties with the nose or sinuses and sense of smell; headaches (when the mind is clogged "like a NYC garbage strike inside the body"); fatigue; eye problems; scanty menstruation; poor circulation headaches due to being stuck in negativity; wakes between 5 a.m. and 7 a.m.; likes or dislikes autumn, spicy food, and the color white. The person's voice sounds sad and weepy.

EMOTIONAL/SPIRITUAL IMBALANCES OF THE COLON:

When this pathway is out of balance, the person may experience the following emotional/spiritual problems: unforgiving, obstinate ("that old battle ax"), stuck, stubborn; a harsh or twisted person, negative thinkers, complainers;

sense of futility or alienation, despair; low self-esteem, think they are shit; live in the past (the past is still alive in them).

TO TREAT THE COLON PATHWAY
➥ TURN TO PAGE 140

WATER

You have chosen to work on the water element. The water element has two pathways associated with it, the bladder and the kidney. This section is designed to give you the information you need to decide if one of those pathways is more important for you than the other.

Please circle or underline any characteristics or symptoms that relate to you on the bladder pathway and then on the kidney pathway. When you are done, select the pathway you want to begin with. Turn to the treatment plan for that pathway and follow the directions. When you are ready, you can work on the other pathway.

If you cannot decide which pathway you want to start with, it is OK to work on both pathways simultaneously. Remember to keep good, clear records of what you do. That way, if you have good results you can duplicate your experience. Also, good records will enable us to gather more information to help others in the future.

After you have worked on the water element for a while, you may feel ready to move onto another element. Feel free to do this. You can always come back to the water element when you need it.

You may want to pay extra special attention to the water element in the season associated with it, winter, or when you are having symptoms related to the water element.

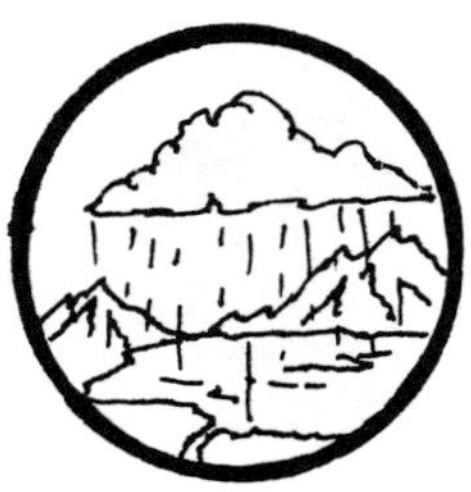

"ORDINARY MIRACLES/EXTRAORDINARY PEOPLE"

LEO'S STORY

I started on October 13, 1993. Within the first two weeks my itching cleared up and my swelling got less. We started with six stings and I worked my way up to twenty-four and eventually dropped down to twenty. My aches and pains cleared up in one or two sessions. I definitely noticed improvement with my bladder problems. Due to my MS, I used to have to go to the bathroom all the time and I had trouble waiting. Now I can hold my urine longer, and the stream is better. All the people at Amber's who are getting bladder stings have been helped by the bees. Also, my hands used to be ice cold all the time and now they are normal.

I have also noticed increased energy. I'm doing more things. I volunteer to work with the bees twice a week. I collect bees for Amber every Friday. It's much easier in the warm weather. In the cold weather I have to warm up the jars with a hair dryer to get the bees to come out. I really enjoy being involved helping everyone with the bees. I fixed Amber's ramp recently and now it won't warp anymore.

I am very excited that one of the people who comes to Amber's house for stings is starting to walk again. He is an inspiration to all of us. One of the best things for me is getting to hang out with other people who are being stung. Everyone shares in each other's successes. It is a real feeling of family. My life has a lot more meaning now.

LEO IS A GODSEND! I DON'T KNOW WHAT I'D DO WITHOUT HIM. HE PITCHES IN WHENEVER HELP IS NEEDED. HE'S A REAL NETWORKER. HE ALWAYS HAS A SMILE AND A JOKE TO SHARE. HE OFTEN DOES MY DISHES. HE IS A VERY IMPORTANT PART OF THIS "STING OPERATION." A.R.

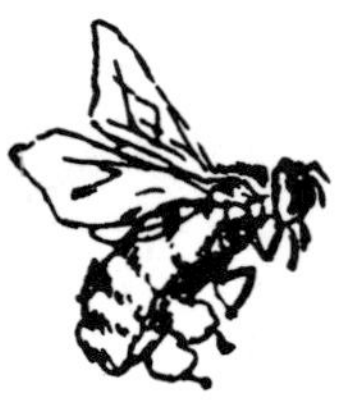

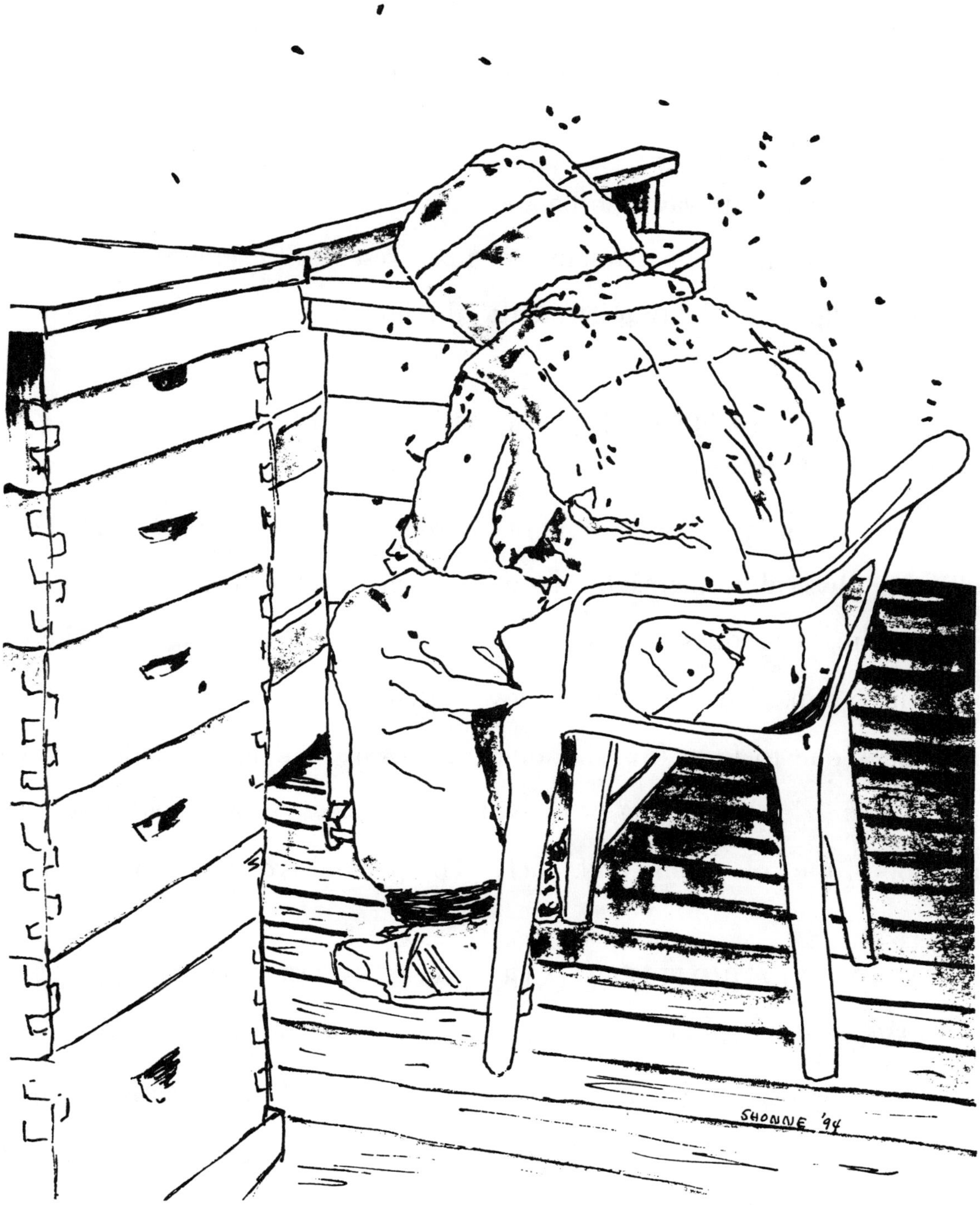

This is Leo Montgomery collecting bees for stinging. "I collect bees for Amber every Friday."

THE BLADDER

Circle or underline any item(s) on this page that you feel relate to you:

POSITIVE QUALITIES:

When this pathway is in balance, the person has the ability to store fluids including urine and thus maintain adequate reserves for emergencies, elasticity, courage, willpower; ability to stretch to the limits, flexible.

PHYSICAL CONDITIONS (ESPECIALLY IN CHILDHOOD) THAT MAY CAUSE OR SIGNAL AN IMBALANCE IN THE BLADDER:

When this pathway is out of balance, the person may experience the following physical problems: feeling tired (burnt out, burning your candle at both ends), feeling a tiredness as if someone has just pulled the plug (often between 3 p.m. and 5 p.m.); "my batteries are low"; environmental illness; lack of flexibility; headaches due to fear, frozen shoulders (frozen with fear); bladder problems; excess fluid (edema) swelling or dehydration; dislikes or likes cold weather, rain, salty foods, the colors blue and black; The person's voice sounds like a groan.

EMOTIONAL/SPIRITUAL IMBALANCES OF THE BLADDER:

When this pathway is out of balance, the person may experience the following emotional/spiritual problems: fear, or lack of fear (Evel Knievel), panic, terror, feeling overwhelmed, "I don't have anything left to give"; hibernates (isolates due to fear), afraid to experience ones emotions; needing to relax and replenish, wants a vacation by the water or to a cold climate; feeling depleted due to a sudden shock; when the fear is so great it's hard to have a relationship, frozen or paralyzed with fear, phobias, living on the edge, taking on the hardest projects and pushing oneself to the limits.

TO TREAT THE BLADDER PATHWAY
➥ TURN TO PAGE 144

THE KIDNEYS

Circle or underline any item(s) on this page that you feel relate to you:

POSITIVE QUALITIES:

When this pathway is in balance, the person may be very energetic; clever, powerful, courageous, peaceful, ambitious, have strong willpower; "goes with the flow"; an inner drive from deep within.

PHYSICAL CONDITIONS (ESPECIALLY IN CHILDHOOD) THAT MAY CAUSE OR SIGNAL AN IMBALANCE IN THE KIDNEY:

When this pathway is out of balance, the person may experience the following physical problems: kidney problems, kidney stones, high fevers that burn up the fluids in the body, for eg., measles; edema (swelling due to too much fluid in the body), or dehydration, urinary problems, nephritis; issues with perspiration, and night sweats; dry eyes or dryness in the body; low back and/or knee pain; joint problems; shortness of breath, listlessness or fatigue; environmental illness; cold limbs; darkish face (especially dark circles around the eyes); headaches due to fear, birth defects or mental retardation; chronic ear aches or deafness; premature white or gray hair, baldness, bone problems, tooth problems; feels better or has problems that are more severe in winter or between 5 p.m. and 7 p.m.; likes or dislikes the colors blue/black, and salty foods. The person's voice sounds like a groan.

EMOTIONAL/SPIRITUAL IMBALANCES OF THE KIDNEY:

When this pathway is out of balance, the person may experience the following emotional/spiritual problems: defects in will power, i.e., addictions, no will to stop smoking or drinking, no ambition; stuck because of fear, terror or panic; giving up due to fear of life, "I just can't do it!," and very deep fears, paranoia or everything becomes the enemy (environmental illness, chemical sensitivity), or a total lack of fear (daredevil).

TO TREAT THE KIDNEY PATHWAY
➡ TURN TO PAGE 151

CHAPTER 7

TREATMENT PLANS

The following treatment plans suggest a number of approaches to selecting sting locations. Now that you have chosen the primary element(s) in which you want to work, these plans will assist you in preparing for a treatment session. According to the Chinese understanding of the meridians, each pathway contains specific points. Each meridian, for example, contains a point representing each element, so that whether the pathway is wood or fire, it will contain a point for all five elements. The element point which is the same as the pathway is a special point called the home element[G] point. Each meridian also contains a series of special points, such as a source point[G], entry/exit points[G], a horary point[G], a junction point[G], and tonification[G] and sedation[G] points. Some pathways also include points known as Windows of the Sky[G] and Spirit[G] points. These points can serve dual purposes on some meridians.

The suggested treatment plans incorporate traditional acupuncture knowledge with my experience in the application of bees to this oriental system of healing. You may want to begin with multiple stings on one pathway; this gives the body a clear instruction, and avoids confusion by trying to do too many things at the same time. This is in accord with the Law of Least Action; while we are tempted to think that more is better, excessive instructions can send mixed messages and detract from simple clarity. As you develop an understanding of the five element system, you will learn to expand your sessions to include a greater number of points which exist in relationship to one another.

Once you've gone past the "itching" stage, feel free to achieve your 15-20 stings by combining acupuncture locations with "trigger points," "nerve meridians," scars, or any of the other suggestions in this book.

Some points are forbidden to sting. These points are forbidden to moxa in traditional acupuncture, which is a technique for heating the point with an herb. Because these points are contraindicated for heat, it is best not to attempt a "bee-acupuncture" treatment. These points, which are marked with an **F**, can be treated with acupressure—pressure applied to the point with the fingertips.

Some points are also located in anatomical sites such that bee stings may be particularly uncomfortable. These points are noted as ones which should be stung "with care." Some points may also itch or swell if you go there too early in your acclimation to the stings. You may want to wait, for example, until you've completed your first month before attempting stings on your hands and feet.

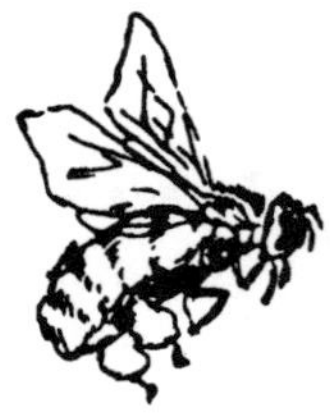

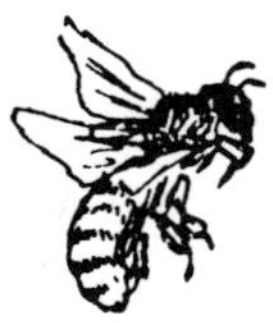

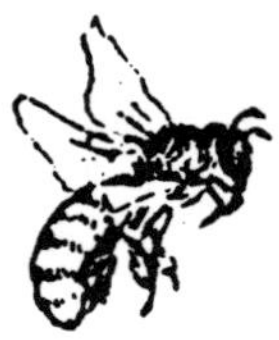

TREATMENT PLAN FOR THE GALL BLADDER PATHWAY

Here is a possible treatment plan to work on the gallbladder (GB) pathway. This plan is immediately followed by point names and locations.

1. If you want to strengthen the GB pathway, you can sting the tonification point (GB-43) or the source point (GB-40).

2. If you want to connect the GB to its paired meridian, the liver (LV), sting yourself on the junction point (GB-37). (See glossary for more information.)

3. You can enhance the effectiveness of your treatment by stinging the home element point (GB-41). This is best done as a horary treatment, which means a treatment on the home element point at the right time of day (11 p.m.—1 a.m.) and or in the right season (spring).

4. If you are having symptoms between 11 p.m.—1 a.m., (i.e., having trouble going to sleep, or waking up at this time every night), then you may want to sting the entry point (GB-1), taking care because this point is close to the eye, and/or exit point (GB-41). Another time to consider stinging the entry/exit points is if you start to feel better and then you feel like you are going backwards. Your symptoms may go away or are alleviated, and then all of a sudden they return again. Instead of getting discouraged, try stinging the entry/exit points!

5. Choose a specific point on the GB based on the name of the point. This is called treating by the spirit of the point. Look at the names of all the points on the GB pathway. Do any of the names jump out at you? What about Bright and Clear (GB 37)? That point is good for seeing things clearly. Do you have trouble with your eyes? Or are you confused? Bright and Clear may be the point for you. Or how about Neglected Muscles (GB 23); does that name bring up thoughts of muscles that have atrophied or are not being used? These are just two examples of some of the points that might speak to you.

6. Try combining any of the above recommendations. "BEE" creative. And remember to keep good records.

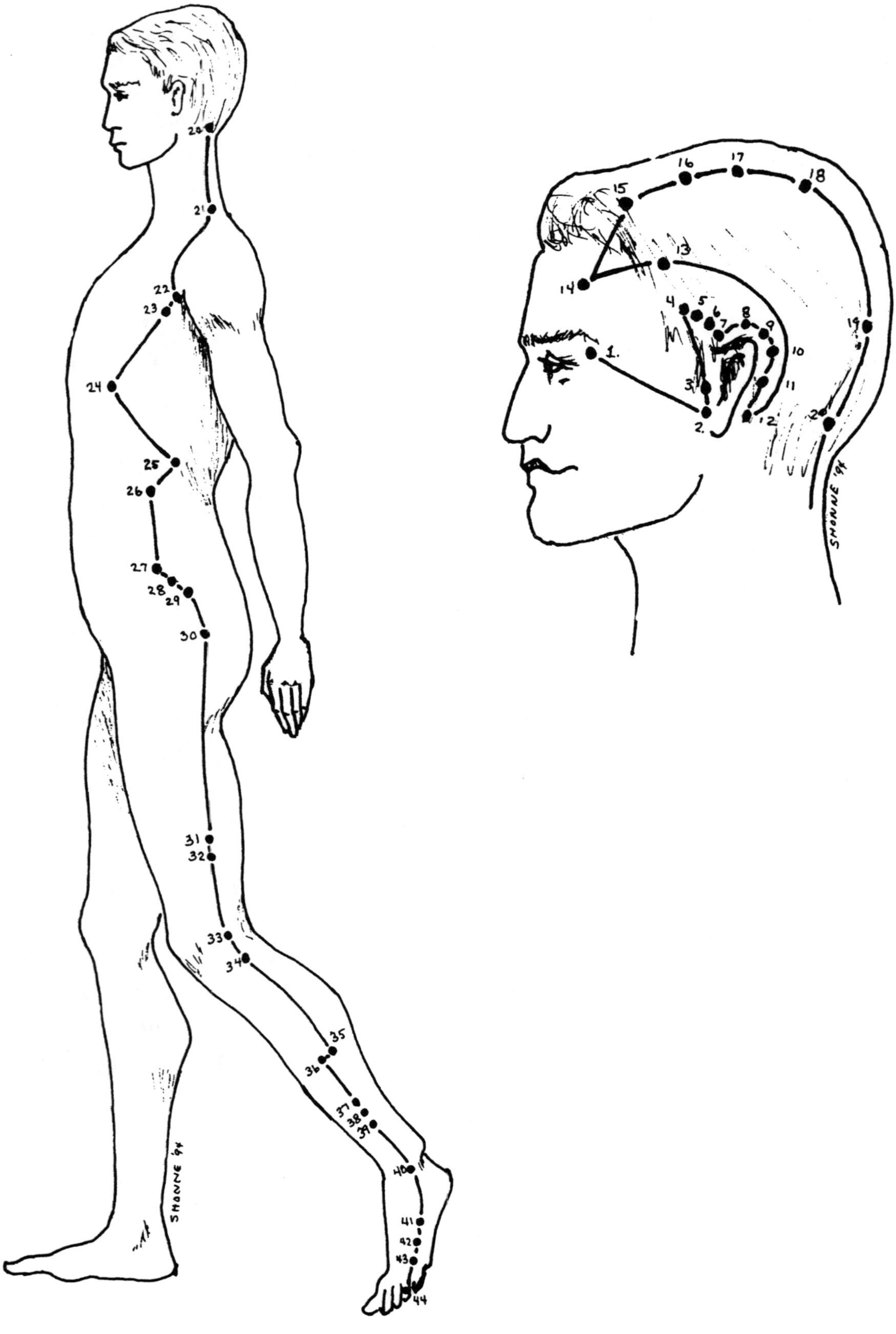

GALL BLADDER PATHWAY

GALL BLADDER PATHWAY (GB)

GB-1 Orbit Bone (entry pt.)(take care because this is close to the eye)

GB-2 Hearing Assembly

GB-3 Upper Pass

GB-4 Forehead Fullness

GB-5 Suspended Skull

GB-6 Suspended Regulator

GB-7 Temporal Hairline Curve

GB-8 Valley Lead

GB-9 Heaven Rushing

GB-10 Floating White

GB-11 Head Porthole Yin

GB-12 Completion Bone

GB-13 Root Spirit

GB-14 Yang White

GB-15 Head Overlooking Tears

GB-16 Eye Window (this is not officially a Window to the Sky but it can be used that way for the whole wood element)

GB-17 Upright Construction

GB-18 Receiving Spirit

GB-19 Brain Hollow

GB-20 Wind Pond (good pt. for muscles; first aid pt: poison)

GB-21 Shoulder Well

GB-22 Armpit Abyss

GB-23 Neglected Muscles

GB-24 Sun and Moon (a good pt. for someone who feels split, opposite polar feelings!)

GB-25 Capital Gate

GB-26 Girdle Vessel

GB-27 Fifth Pivot (good pt. for hip problems and balance)

GB-28 Binding Path (good pt. for hip problems and balance)

GB-29 Dwelling in the Bone (good pt. for hip problems and balance)

GB-30 Jumping Round (first aid pt: fractures and sprains)

GB-31 Wind Market

GB-32 Middle Ditch

GB-33 Knee Yang Joint

GB-34 Yang Mound Spring (earth pt. and assembling pt. of tendons, muscles; lack of coordination and paralysis, knee and ankle problems)

GB-35 Yang Crossing (good for chest, legs, feet, muscles)

GB-36 Outer Mound (a good pt. for intense dislike of wind)

GB-37 Bright and Clear (junction pt. and good pt. for eyes, paralysis, drug users, rigidity and spasm, coordinating muscles and tendons, and for those who are having trouble standing)

GB-38 Yang Support (fire and sedation pts.)

GB-39 Severed Bone (assembling pt. of marrow and meeting pt. of the bladder, gallbladder and stomach pathway; this pt. is good for bone marrow and cortisone production)

GB-40 Wilderness Mound (source pt., good spirit pt. for getting a perspective on your life; first aid pt: food poisoning, poison, lack of co-ordination, swelling and sighing)

GB-41 Foot Overlooking Tears (wood, home element, exit and horary pts., 11 p.m.—1 a.m. This is a pt. related to getting above angry tears; a good pt. for rheumatism.)

GB-42 Earth Five-Fold

GB-43 Valiant Stream (water and tonification pts., good pt. for puffy face, too much or too little water; this point is good to cool down anger and violence)

GB-44 Foot Hole Yin (metal pt., good pt. for inability to move arms and legs due to pain, inability to speak and bend knees, insomnia)

TREATMENT PLAN FOR THE LIVER PATHWAY (LV)

Here is a possible treatment plan to work on the liver (LV) pathway. This plan is immediately followed by point names and locations.

1. If you want to strengthen the LV pathway, you can sting the tonification point (LV-8) or the source point (LV-3).

2. If you want to connect the LV to its paired meridian the gall bladder (GB), sting yourself on the junction point (LV-5). (See glossary for more information.)

3. You can enhance the effectiveness of your treatment by stinging the home element point (LV-1). This is best done as a horary treatment, which means a treatment on the home element point at the right time of day (1 a.m.—3 a.m.) and/or in the right season (spring).

4. If you are having symptoms between 1 a.m.—3 a.m. (i.e., having trouble falling asleep then, or waking up at that time every night), then you may want to sting the entry point (LV-1) and/or the exit points (LV-13 and LV-14). Another reason to consider stinging the entry/exit points is if you start to feel better and then you feel like you are going backwards. Your symptoms may go away or are alleviated, and then all of a sudden they return again. Instead of getting discouraged, try stinging the entry/exit points!

5. Choose a specific point on the LV based on the name of the point. This is called treating by the spirit of the point. Look at the names of all the points on the LV pathway. Do any of the names jump out at you? What about Chapter Gate (LV-13)? This is all about starting a new chapter in your life. Does that sound like you? Or how about Gate of Hope (LV-14)? Are you feeling depressed or hopeless? Do you feel like nothing is ever going to change? These are just two examples of some of the points on the LV that might speak to you.

6. Try combining any of the above recommendations. "BEE" creative. And remember to keep good records.

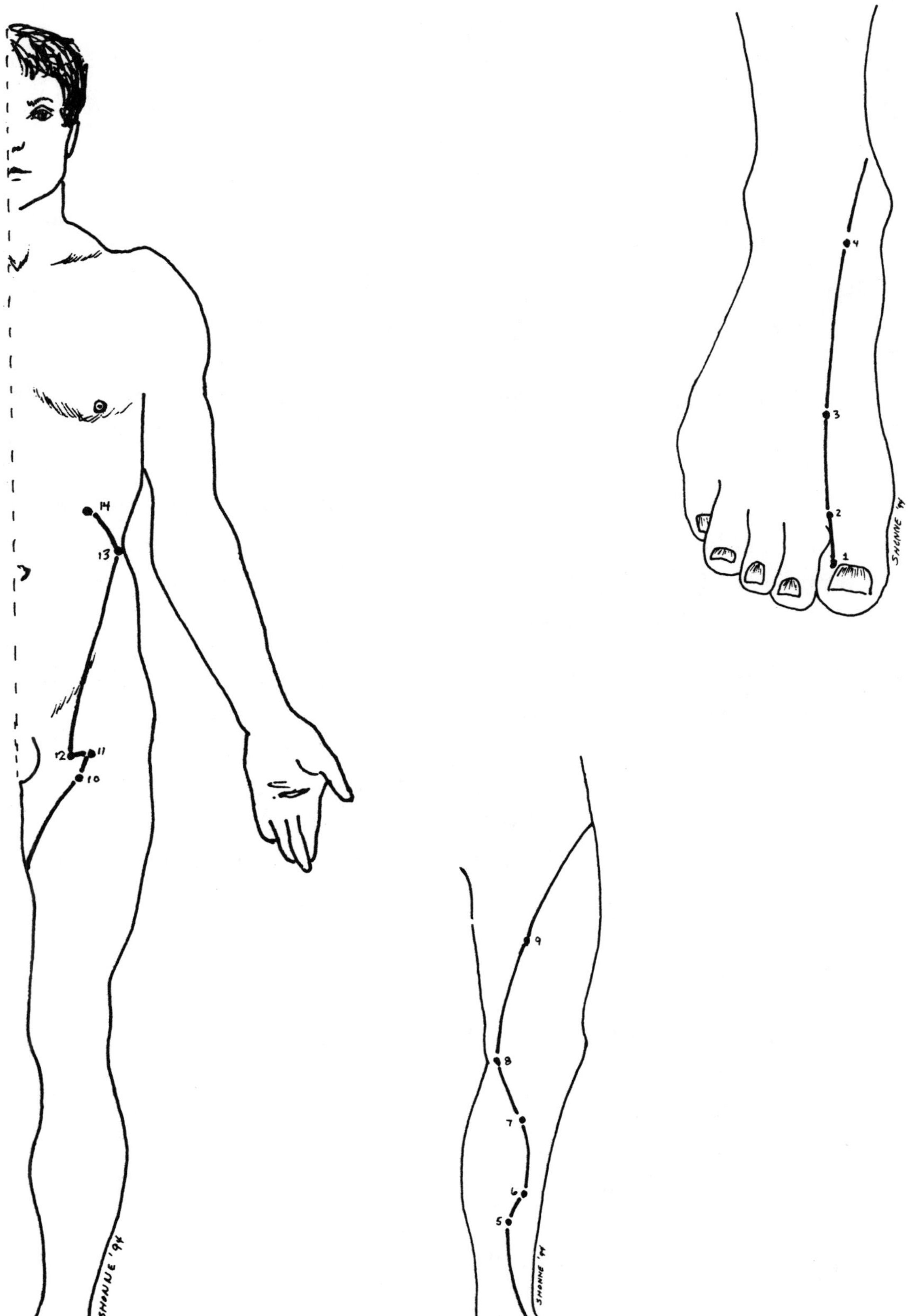

14
13
12
11
10
SHONNE '94
4
3
2
1
9
8
7
6
5

LIVER PATHWAY (LV)

LV-1 Great Esteem (wood, home element, entry, and horary pts., 1 a.m.—3 a.m.)

LV-2 Moving Between (fire and sedation pts., first aid pt: cramps, spasms)

LV-3 Happy Calm (earth and source pts., as well as a good pt. for getting toxins out of the body. This is a good pt. for allergies.)

LV-4 Middle Seal (metal pt. and a very good spiritual pt. for finding your identity; good pt. for cold legs and feet, muscle spasms, paralysis)

LV-5 Insect Ditch (junction pt. and a center of energy; this point is good if you feel like you are restless as if you have "ants in your pants"; a helpful point if you are unable to walk or stand; this is also good for cramps, abdominal pain, menstrual problems)

LV-6 Middle Capital (center of energy; first aid pt: cramps, spasms, and urine retention, also weakness and inability to stand, paralysis)

LV-7 Knee Joint (good for knee disorders)

LV-8 Spring at the Bend (water and tonification pts., a good pt. for urinary problems, fear, depression, anger, irritation, jealousy)

LV-9 Yin Wrapping

LV-10 Five Miles

LV-11 Yin Corner

LV-12 Urgent Pulse

LV-13 Chapter Gate (exit pt., good for starting a new chapter in your life)

LV-14 Gate of Hope (exit pt. and good pt. for depression, despair and feeling hopeless)

TREATMENT PLAN FOR HEART PATHWAY

Here is a possible treatment plan to work on the heart (H) pathway. This plan is immediately followed by point names and locations.

1. If you want to strengthen the H pathway, you can sting the tonification point (H-9) or the source point (H-7).

2. If you want to connect the H to its paired meridian the small intestine (SI), sting yourself on the junction point (H-5). (See glossary for more information.)

3. You can enhance the effectiveness of your treatment by stinging the home element point (H-8). This is best done as a horary treatment, which means a treat on the home element point at the right time of day (11 a.m.—1 p.m.) and/or in the right season (summer).

4. If you are having symptoms between 11 a.m.—1 p.m. (i.e., feeling tired or feeling depressed) you may want to sting the entry point (H-1) and/or the exit point (H-9). Another reason to consider stinging the entry/exit points is if you start to feel better and then you feel like you are going backwards. Your symptoms may go away or are alleviated, and then all of a sudden they return again. Instead of getting discouraged, try stinging the entry/exit points!

5. Choose a specific point on the H based on the name of the point. This is called treating by the spirit of the point. Look at the names of all the points on the H pathway. Do any of the names jump out at you? What about Spirit Path? (H-4) That is a point where you go to find your spiritual path. Or how about a point that will get to the heart of the matter, Penetrating Inside (H-5)? These are just two examples of some of the points on the H that might speak to you.

6. Try combining any of the above recommendations. "BEE" creative. And remember to keep good records.

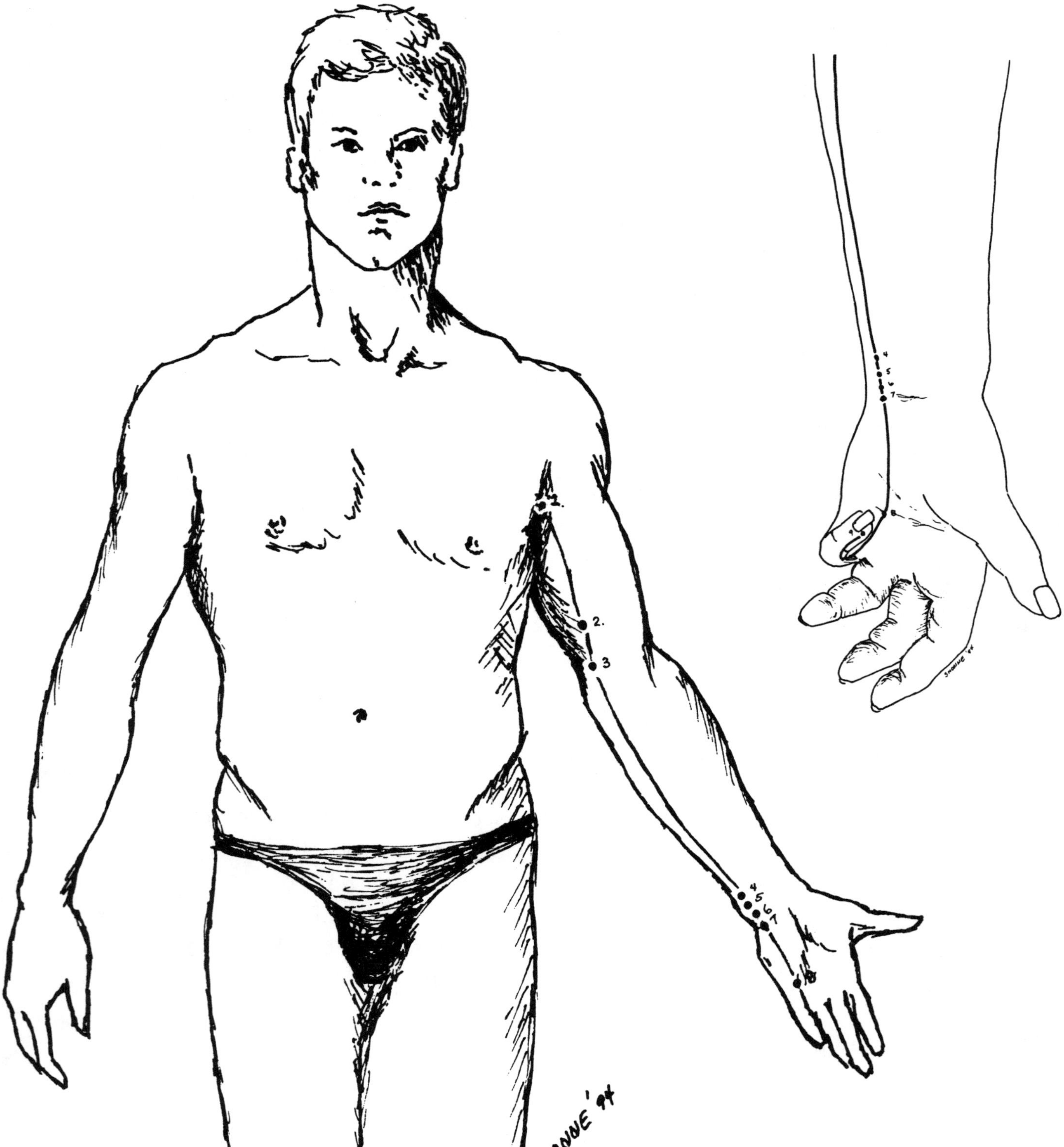

HEART PATHWAY

HEART PATHWAY (H)

H-1 Utmost Source (entry pt.)

H-2 Blue-Green Spirit

H-3 Lesser Sea (water pt.)

H-4 Spirit Path (metal pt.)

H-5 Penetrating Inside (junction pt.)

H-6 Yin Mound

H-7 Spirit Gate (earth, sedation, and source pts.)

H-8 Lesser Mansion (fire, home element, and horary pts., 11 a.m.—1 p.m.)

H-9 Lesser Surge (wood, tonification, and exit pts.)

TREATMENT PLAN FOR THE SMALL INTESTINE

Here is a possible treatment plan to work on the small intestine (SI) pathway. This plan is immediately followed by point names and locations.

1. If you want to strengthen the SI pathway, you can sting the tonification point (SI-3) or the source point (SI-4).

2. If you want to connect the SI to its paired meridian the heart (H), sting yourself on the junction point (SI-7). (See glossary for more information.)

3. You can enhance the effectiveness of your treatment by stinging the home element point (SI-5). This is best done as a horary treatment, which means a treatment on the home element point at the right time of day (1 p.m.—3 p.m.) and/or in the right season (summer).

4. If you are having symptoms between 1 p.m.—3 p.m. (i.e., feeling tired or having trouble concentrating), then you may want to sting the entry point (SI-1) and/or the exit point (SI-19). Another reason to consider stinging the entry/exit points is if you start to feel better and then you feel like you are going backwards. Your symptoms may go away or are alleviated, and then all of a sudden they return again. Instead of getting discouraged, try stinging the entry/exit points!

5. Choose a specific point on the SI based on the name of the point. This is called treating by the spirit of the point. Look at the names of all the points on the SI pathway. Do any of the names jump out at you? What about Nourishing the Old (SI-6)? This point helps you let go of what you don't need from the past, but lets you treasure what was good. This is just one example of some of the points on the SI that might speak to you.

6. Also consider the possibility of stinging a Window of the Sky. The SI has two of them: (SI-16) and (SI-17). Windows of the Sky are traditionally done when you want to bring the body, mind and spirit back into balance.

7. Try combining any of the above recommendations. "BEE" creative. And remember to keep good records.

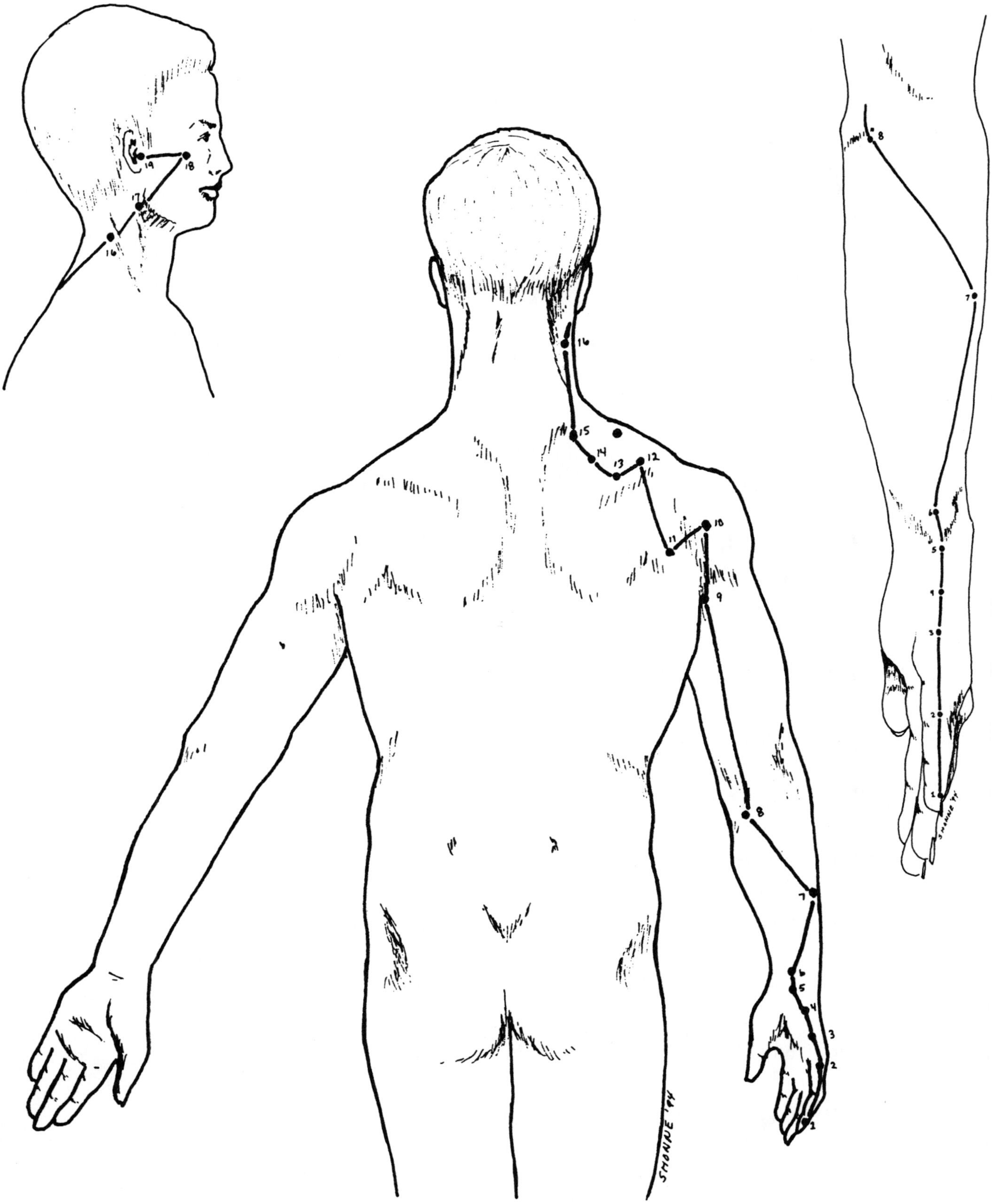

SMALL INTESTINE PATHWAY

SMALL INTESTINE PATHWAY (SI)

SI-1 Lesser Marsh (metal and entry pts.)

SI-2 Front Valley (water pt.)

SI-3 Back Ravine (wood and tonification pts.)

SI-4 Wrist Bone (source pt.)

SI-5 Yang Valley (fire, home element, and horary pts., 1 p.m.—3 p.m., good pt. for tinnitus and Bell's Palsy)

SI-6 Nourishing the Old (a good spirit point for helping let go of things from the past that you don't need, yet treasure the good things)

SI-7 Branch to the Correct (junction pt.)

SI-8 Small Sea (earth and sedation pts.)

SI-9 True Shoulder

SI-10 Shoulder Blade

SI-11 Celestial Gathering

SI-12 Grasping the Wind

SI-13 Crooked Wall

SI-14 Outside the Shoulder Correspondence

SI-15 Middle of the Shoulder Correspondence

SI-16 Celestial Window (Window of the Sky)

SI-17 Heavenly Appearance (Window of the Sky)

F SI-18 Cheek Bone-Hole (can use acupressure)

SI-19 Listening Palace (exit pt.)

The **F** refers to points which are forbidden to sting.

TREATMENT PLAN FOR HEART PROTECTOR PATHWAY

Here is a possible treatment plan to work on the heart protector (HP) pathway. This plan is immediately followed by point names and locations.

1. If you want to strengthen the HP pathway, you can sting the tonification point (HP-9) or the source point (HP-7).

2. If you want to connect the HP to its paired meridian the three heater (TH), sting yourself on the junction point (HP-6). (See glossary for more information.)

3. You can enhance the effectiveness of your treatment by stinging the horary point (HP-8) at the right time of day (7 p.m.—9 p.m.) and/or in the right season (summer).

4. If you are having symptoms between 7 p.m.—9 p.m. (i.e., feeling tired or feeling depressed) you may want to sting the entry point (HP-1 for men/HP-2 for women) and/or the exit point (HP-8). Another reason to consider stinging the entry/exit points is if you start to feel better and then you feel like you are going backwards. Your symptoms may go away or are alleviated, and then all of a sudden they return again. Instead of getting discouraged, try stinging the entry/exit points!

5. Choose a specific point on the HP based on the name of the point. This is called treating by the spirit of the point. Look at the names of all the points on the HP pathway. Do any of the names jump out at you? What about Palace of Weariness (HP-8)? That is a palace where you go to rejuvenate yourself. Or how about Inner Frontier Gate (HP-6)? This opens the gate to communicate with others on a more intimate level. These are just two examples of some of the points on the H that might speak to you.

6. You might want to consider stinging a Window of the Sky (HP-1 for men and HP-2 for women). This will bring the body, mind and spirit together.

7. Try combining any of the above recommendations. "BEE" creative. And remember to keep good records.

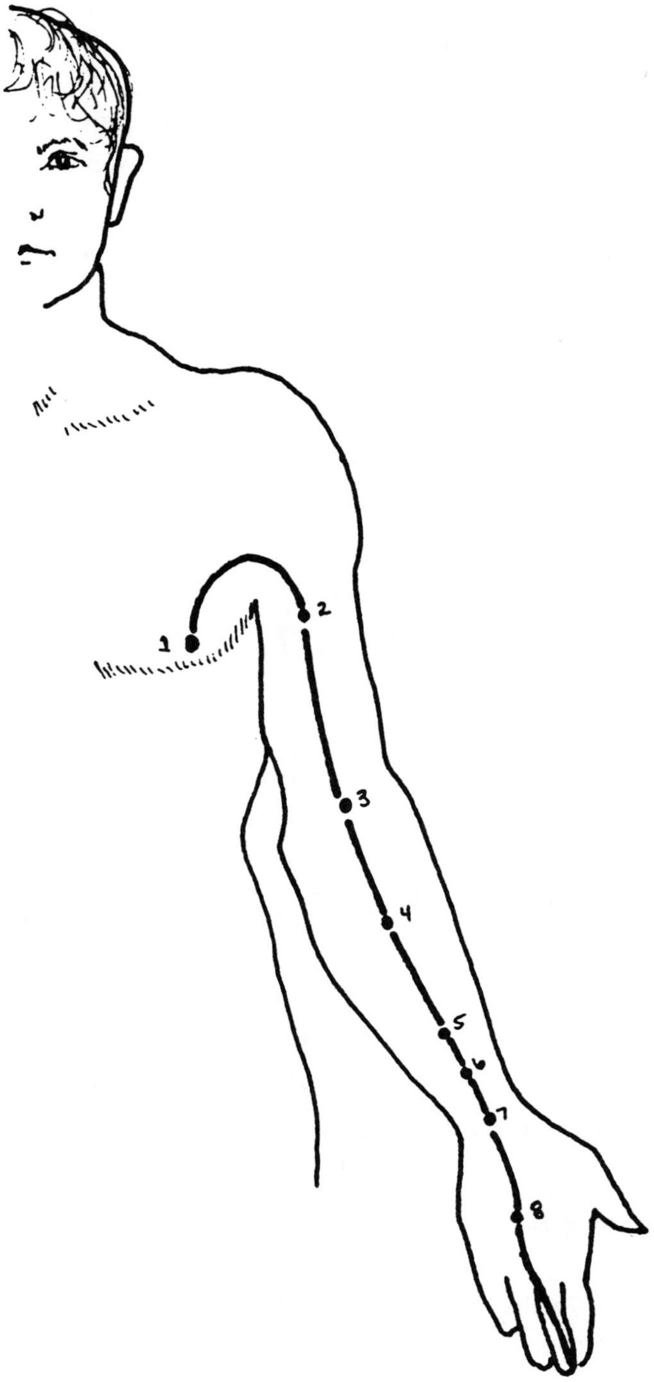
1
2
3
4
5
6
7
8

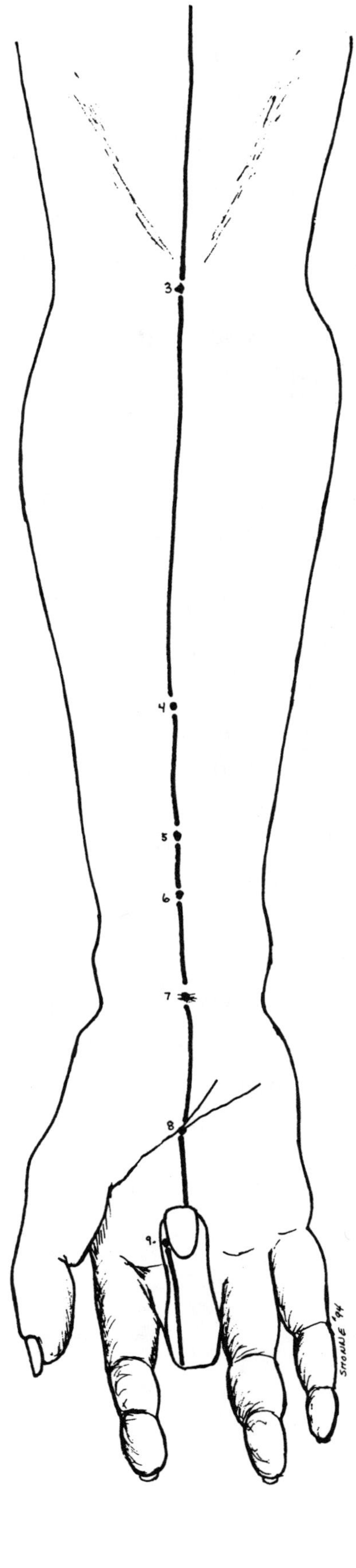
3
4
5
6
7
8
9

HEART PROTECTOR PATHWAY (HP)

HP-1 Celestial Pool (entry pt. for men and Window of the Sky)
F in women

HP-2 Celestial Spring (entry pt. for women and Window of the Sky)

HP-3 Marsh at the Bend (water pt., a good pt. for someone who has a fear of water and of meeting people)

HP-4 Gate of *Ch'i* Reserve (a good pt. for a patient who feels that he or she has no energy and can't go on, an excellent pt. for a person who is suffering on the mental level)

HP-5 Intermediary Courier (metal pt., good pt. for grief in the heart, turning to God, a good pt. for food lying heavy in stomach)

HP-6 Inner Frontier Gate (junction pt., good point for anxiety and depression)

HP-7 Great Mound (earth, sedation and source pts. for fevers with much weariness, for people who are very sad; lack of stability and lack of control)

HP-8 Palace of Weariness (fire, home element, exit and horary pts., 7 p.m.—9 p.m., with this point closed, it is hard to have a successful marriage; lack of warmth, and lack of tolerance, asthma; a good point for those who are trying to be warm and loving, and yet feel they want to give up, and then become sad, miserable, or rigid)

HP-9 Central Hub (wood and tonification pts., first aid pt: anxiety and resuscitation, varicose veins, epilepsy)

The **F** refers to points which are forbidden to sting.

TREATMENT PLAN FOR THE THREE HEATER PATHWAY (TH)

Here is a possible treatment plan to work on the three heater (TH) pathway. This plan is immediately followed by point names and locations.

1. If you want to strengthen the TH pathway, you can sting the tonification point (TH-3) or the source point (TH-4).

2. If you want to connect the TH to its paired meridian the heart protector (HP), sting yourself on the junction point (TH-5). (See glossary for more.)

3. You can enhance the effectiveness of your treatment by stinging the home element point (TH-6). This is best done as a horary treatment, which means a treatment on the home element point at the right time of day (9 p.m.—11 p.m.) and/or in the right season (summer).

4. If you are having symptoms between 9 p.m.—11 p.m. (i.e., having trouble falling asleep then, or feeling depressed), then you may want to sting the entry point (TH-1) and/or the exit point (TH-22). Another reason to consider stinging the entry/exit points is if you start to feel better and then you feel like you are going backwards. Your symptoms may go away or are alleviated, and then all of a sudden they return again. Instead of getting discouraged, try stinging the entry/exit points!

5. Choose a specific point on the TH based on the name of the point. This is called treating by the spirit of the point. Look at the names of all the points on the TH pathway. Do any of the names jump out? What about Pure Cold Abyss (TH-11)? Does that sound like you? Do you ever feel really cold and can't get warm? This is just one example of some of the points that might speak to you.

6. You also might want to consider doing a Window of the Sky (TH-16). This is a good point for bringing the body, mind and spirit together. If you are seeking a breakthrough, this may be a good point for you. It is also located behind and just below the mastoid process of the ear, so this is a good place to sting for balance, hearing problems, vision and mental clarity.

7. Try combining any of the above recommendations. "BEE" creative. And remember to keep good records.

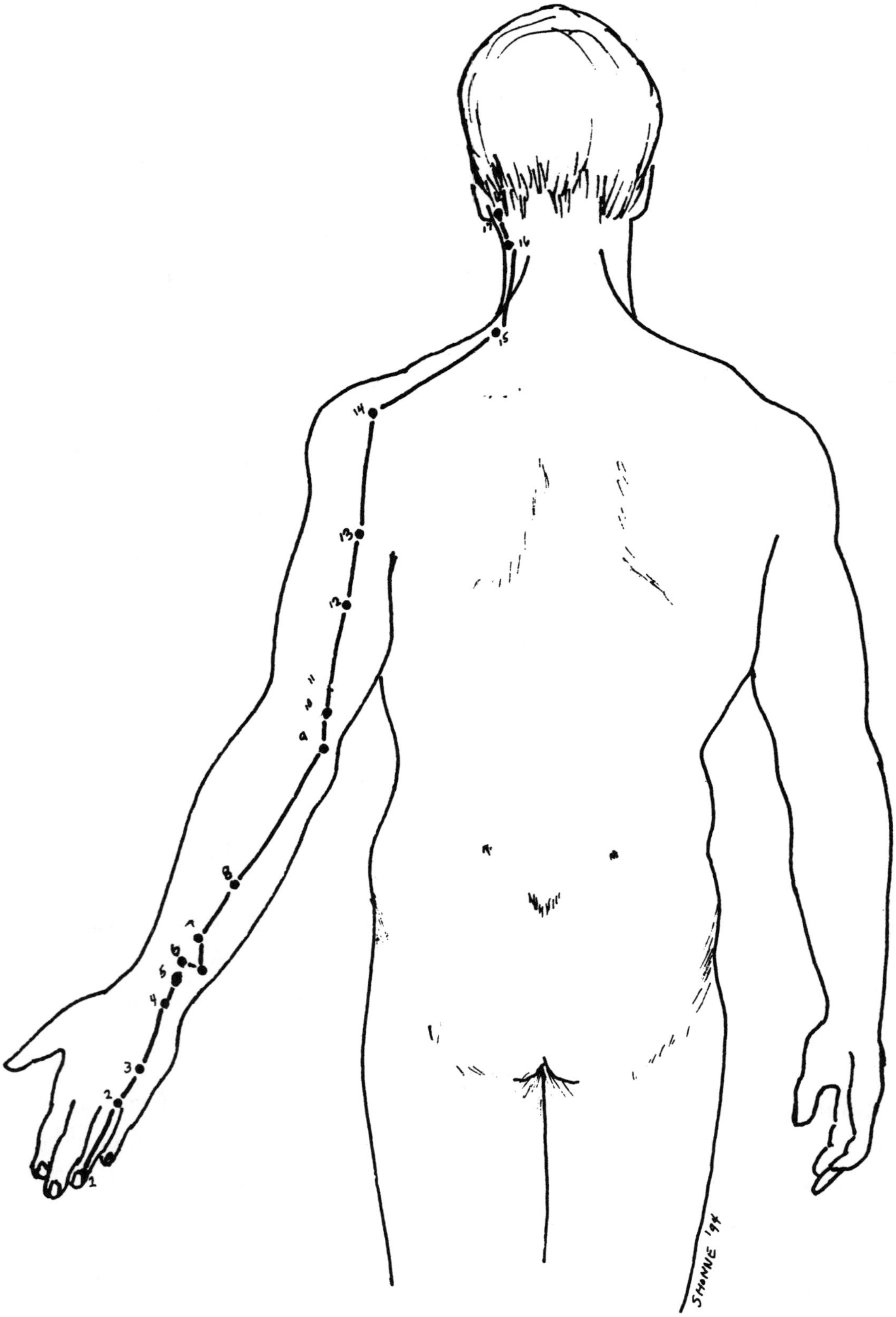

THREE HEATER PATHWAY

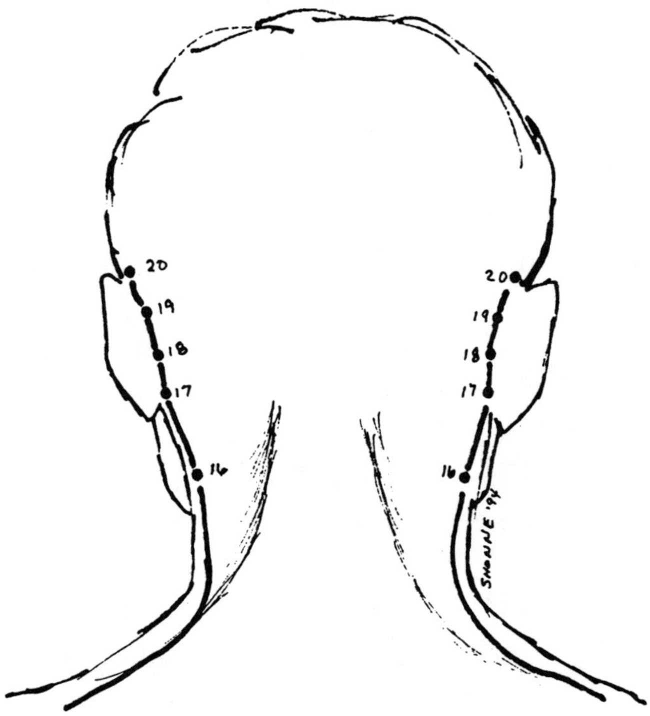
20
19
18
17
16
20
19
18
17
16
SHONNE '94

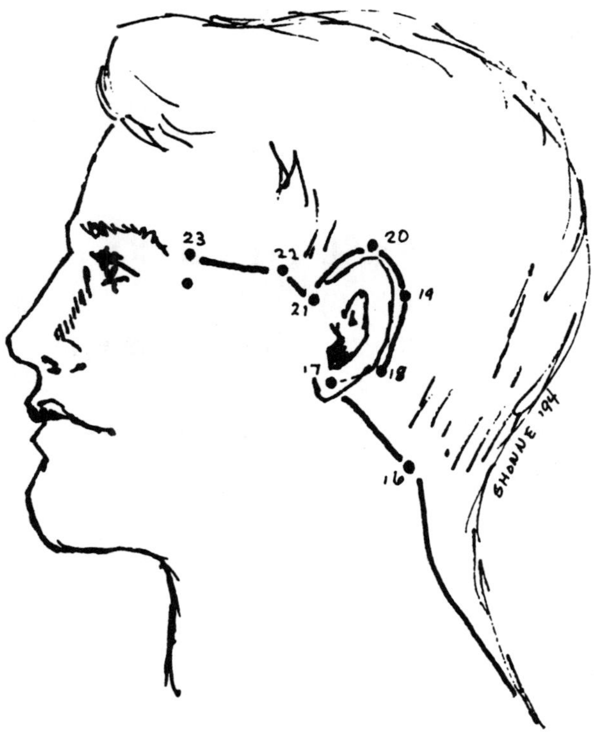
23
22
21
20
19
17
18
16
SHONNE '94

THREE HEATER PATHWAY (TH)

TH-1 Rushing the Frontier Gate (metal and entry pts., good pt. for coldness, rigidity, trouble with elbow, unable to raise forearm, frozen shoulder, tennis elbow, numbness)

TH-2 Humor Gate (water pt., good pt. for cold or hot hands and feet, tinnitus, eyes red and painful, mind wanders)

TH-3 Central Islet (wood and tonification pts.; first aid pt: exhaustion, dizziness and lack of balance)

TH-4 Yang Pool (source pt., good pt. for inability to grasp and hold objects, to raise shoulder and bend fingers, also good for improved hearing)

TH-5 Outer Frontier Gate (junction pt., good pt. for difficulty hearing and headaches, ulcers, patient feels that people are a "pain in the neck"; it is a good point for reaching out to others)

TH-6 Branch Ditch (fire, home element, and horary pts., 9 p.m.—11 p.m., good for arthritis and rheumatic conditions)

TH-7 Assembly of Ancestors (a good pt. if you are wondering "Where do I go from here?")

TH-8 Three Yang Connection (meeting pt. for SI, TH and CO; this is good for lack of coordination, pain in the loins, eye diseases, keep this point in mind for a situation when the "body doesn't wish to move")

TH-9 Four Rivers (good pt. for eye disorders, problems with forearm and elbow)

TH-10 Celestial Well (earth and sedation pts.)

TH-11 Pure Cold Abyss

TH-12 Relax and Joy

TH-13 Shoulder Meeting

TH-14 Shoulder Bone Hole

TH-15 Celestial Bone-Hole (first aid pt: colds)

TH-16 Heavenly Window (Window of the Sky)

TH-17 Wind Screen

TH-18 Spasm Vessel

TH-19 Skull Breathing

TH-20 Small Angle of Ear

TH-21 Ear Gate

TH-22 Harmony Bone-Hole (exit pt.)

F TH-23 Silk Bamboo Hollow (can use acupressure)

The F refers to points which are forbidden to sting.

TREATMENT PLAN FOR THE STOMACH PATHWAY (ST)

Here is a possible treatment plan to work on the stomach (ST) pathway. This plan is immediately followed by point names and locations.

1. If you want to strengthen the ST pathway, you can sting the tonification point (ST-41) or the source point (ST-42).

2. If you want to connect the ST to its paired meridian the spleen (SP), sting yourself on the junction point (ST-40). (See glossary for more information.)

3. You can enhance the effectiveness of your treatment by stinging the home element point (ST-36). This is best done as a horary treatment, which means a treatment on the home element point at the right time of day (7 a.m.—9 a.m.) and/or in the right season (late summer).

4. If you are having symptoms between 7 a.m.—9 a.m. (i.e., having trouble getting up and getting going, nauseated, or feeling sluggish), then you may want to do acupressure on the entry point (ST-1). This point is forbidden to bee sting, though you can sting the exit point (ST-42). Another reason to consider going to the entry/exit points is if you start to feel better and then you feel like you are going backwards. Your symptoms may go away or are alleviated, and then all of a sudden they return again. Instead of getting discouraged, try treating the entry/exit points!

5. Choose a specific point on the ST based on the name of the point. This is called treating by the spirit of the point. Look at the names of all the points on the ST pathway. Do any of the names jump out at you? What about Hard Bargain (ST-45)? Do you feel like your life is very difficult and it's not fair? Or how about Leg Three Miles (ST-36)? This is a very famous first aid point. It is especially good for nausea, morning sickness, travel sickness. But this point also has another meaning on a spirit level. It is a good point for people who go the extra mile for others, but not for themselves. It's a good point for bringing nurturing and compassion to some one who needs it. These are just two examples of some of the points on the ST that might speak to you.

6. You may want to consider a Window of the Sky, People Welcome (ST-9). Remember that Windows bring the body, mind and spirit together. This is a good point for helping someone let people in to their lives and to open up. Since this point is forbidden for bee stings, you will need to use acupressure only.

7. Try combining any of the above recommendations. "BEE" creative. And remember to keep good records.

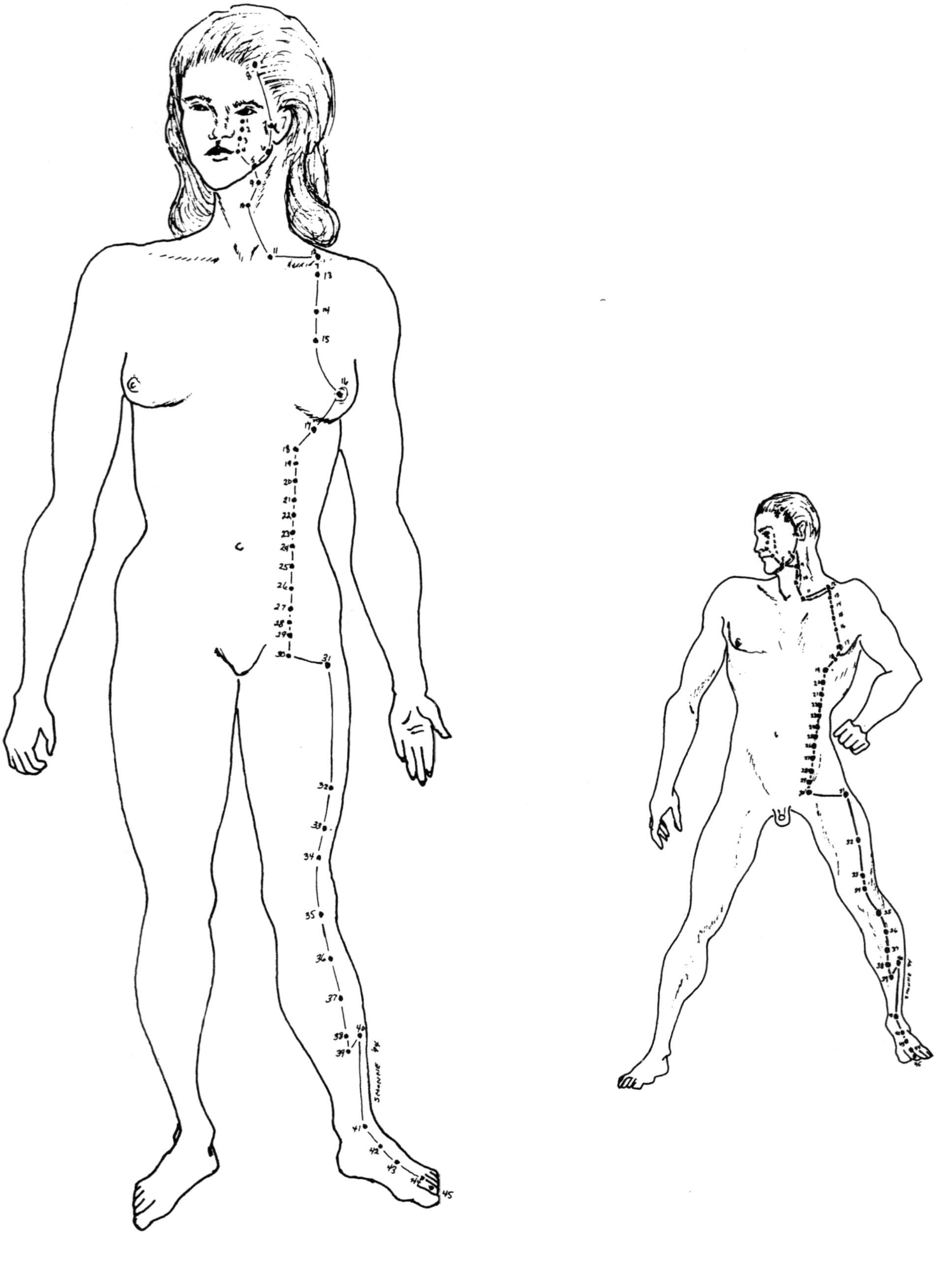

STOMACH PATHWAY

STOMACH PATHWAY (ST)

F ST-1 Receive Tears, Tear Container (entry pt.)(use acupressure only)

F ST-2 Four Whites (use acupressure only)

ST-3 Great Bone-Hole

ST-4 Earth Granary

ST-5 Great Welcome

ST-6 Jaw Bone

ST-7 Below the Joint

ST-8 Head Corner

F ST-9 People Welcome (Window to the Sky. This is a very good spirit pt. for those who need to let people into their lives!)(use acupressure only)

ST-10 Water Rushing Out

ST-11 *Ch'i* Cottage (this is a good pt. for energy)

ST-12 Broken Bowl (this spirit pt. is very good for people who feel like their spirit was broken in childhood. They feel like they are Humpty Dumpty, who can't be put back together again)

ST-13 *Ch'i* Door (a door to energy)

ST-14 Storehouse

ST-15 Roof

ST-16 Breast Window

The **F** refers to points which are forbidden to sting.

ST-16 Breast Window

F ST-17 Center of the Breasts (use acupressure only)

ST-18 Root of the Breasts

ST-19 Not at Ease (Good pt. for anxiety)

ST-20 Receiving Fullness

ST-21 Bridge Gate

ST-22 Border Gate

ST-23 Great Oneness (this is a great pt. for those who feel disconnected from others and the universe)

ST-24 Lubrication Food Gate (this is a good pt. for difficulty with food digestion)

ST-25 Celestial Pivot (Internal Dragon pt. and the place within all of us where we meet God)

ST-26 Outside Mound

ST-27 Great Gigantic

ST-28 Water Path

ST-29 The Return

ST-30 *Ch'i* Rushing (this is a Sea of Nourishment)

ST-31 Thigh Border

The F refers to points which are forbidden to sting.

ST-32 Prostrate Hare (Internal Dragon pt. and a good pt. for exhaustion, like a rabbit lying by the side of the road)

ST-33 Yin Market

ST-34 Beam Mound

ST-35 Calf's Nose

ST-36 Leg Three Miles (earth, home element, and horary pts., 7 a.m.—9 a.m.; first aid pt: indigestion, fainting and morning sickness. This point is very famous because it is also a Sea of Nourishment and a center of energy.)

ST-37 Upper Great Void

ST-38 Branch Opening (this is a good spirit pt. to create an opening for new ideas or actions! Also good for weakness of legs, inability to move limbs and cold limbs.)

ST-39 Lower Great Void (good for hair coming out in handfuls, rheumatism and arthritis)

ST-40 Abundant Splendor (junction pt. and good spirit pt. for abundance)

ST-41 Released Stream (fire and tonification pts. and Internal Dragon pt.; good for rheumatism and gout)

ST-42 Surging Yang (source and exit pts.)

ST-43 Sunken Valley (wood pt. and a spirit point for a feeling of sinking in quicksand)

ST-44 Inner Courtyard (water pt.)

ST-45 Hard Bargain (metal and sedation pts.; first aid: hangover)

TREATMENT PLAN FOR THE SPLEEN PATHWAY (SP)

Here is a possible treatment plan to work on the spleen (SP) pathway. This plan is immediately followed by point names and locations.

1. If you want to strengthen the SP pathway, you can sting the tonification point (SP-2) or the source point (SP-3).

2. If you want to connect the SP to its paired meridian the stomach (ST), sting yourself on the junction point (SP-4). (See glossary for more information.)

3. You can enhance the effectiveness of your treatment by stinging the home element point (SP-3). This is best done as a horary treatment, which means a treatment on the home element point at the right time of day (9 a.m.— 11 a.m.) and/or in the right season (late summer).

4. If you are having symptoms between 9 a.m.—11 a.m. (i.e., having trouble staying wake, feeling sluggish or depressed), then you may want to sting the entry point (SP-1) and/or the exit point (SP-21). Another reason to consider stinging the entry/exit points is if you start to feel better and then you feel like you are going backwards. Your symptoms may go away or are alleviated, and then all of a sudden they return again. Instead of getting discouraged, try stinging the entry/exit points!

5. Choose a specific point on the SP based on the name of the point. This is called treating by the spirit of the point. Look at the names of all the points on the SP pathway. Do any of the names jump out at you? What about Leaky Valley (SP-7)? Do you ever feel like your energy is leaking out of you? Or how about Earth Motivator (SP-8)? Are you feeling depressed and are you having trouble motivating yourself to do anything? These are just two examples of some of the points on the SP that might speak to you.

6. Try combining any of the above recommendations. "BEE" creative. And remember to keep good records.

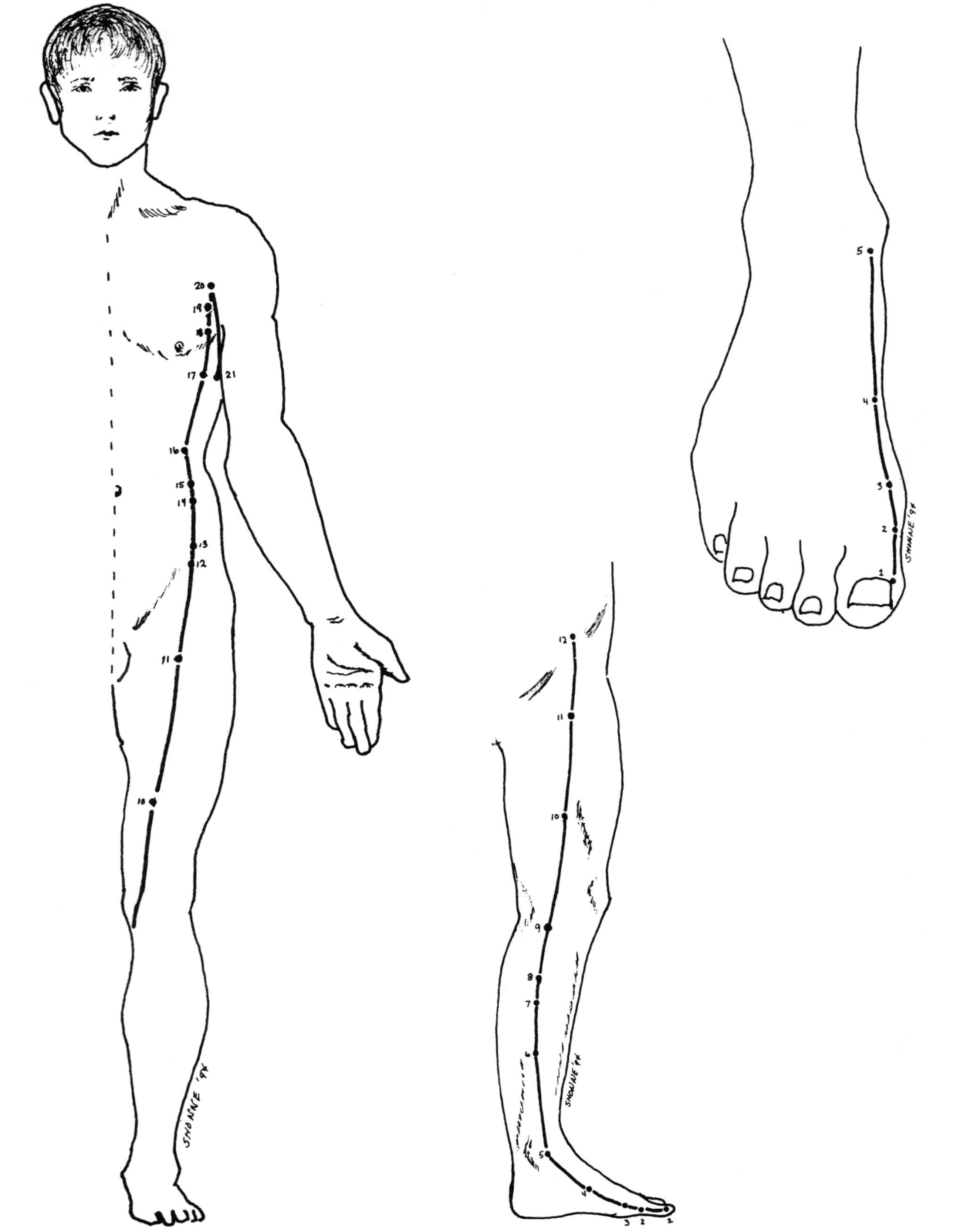

SPLEEN PATHWAY

SPLEEN PATHWAY (SP)

SP-1 Hidden White (wood and entry pts.)

SP-2 Great Metropolis (fire and tonification pts.; first aid pt: fractures and spasms, limbs feel heavy, cold hands and feet)

SP-3 Supreme White, also called "The Mother Within Us that Never Dies" (earth, home element, source and horary pts., 9 a.m.—11 a.m.)

SP-4 Yellow Emperor Prince's Grandson (junction pt. This pt. cured the grandson of the Prince, therefore it may cure you!)

SP-5 Merchant Mound (metal and sedation pts.)

SP-6 Three Yin Intersection (center of energy and a meeting pt. of the Spleen, Kidney and Liver pathways, good for insomnia and depression)

SP-7 Leaky Valley

SP-8 Earth Motivator (this pt. gets the earth moving)

SP-9 Yin Mound Spring (water pt.)

SP-10 Sea of Blood

SP-11 Basket Gate

SP-12 Surging Gate

SP-13 Official Residence

SP-14 Abdomen Knot (a good pt. for knots in the abdomen)

SP-15 Great Horizontal

SP-16 Abdomen Sorrow (this is a spirit pt. for sorrow that is so deep it feels like it goes down to the core of your being)

SP-17 Food Drain

SP-18 Celestial Ravine

SP-19 Chest Village

SP-20 Encircling Glory

SP-21 Great Enveloping (exit pt. and spirit pt. for feeling nurtured and enveloped by motherly love and compassion)

TREATMENT PLAN FOR THE LUNG PATHWAY (L)

Here is a possible treatment plan to work on the lung (L) pathway. This plan is immediately followed by point names and locations.

1. If you want to strengthen the L pathway, you can sting the tonification point (L-9) or the source point (L-9).

2. If you want to connect the L to its paired meridian the colon (CO), sting yourself on the junction point (L-7). (See glossary for more information.)

3. You can enhance the effectiveness of your treatment by stinging the home element point (L-8). This is best done as a horary treatment, which means a treatment on the home element point at the right time of day (3 a.m.—5 a.m.) and/or in the right season (autumn).

4. If you are having symptoms between 3 a.m.—5 a.m. (i.e., waking up at that time every night), then you may want to sting the entry point (L-1) and/or the exit point (L-7). Another reason to consider stinging the entry/exit points is if you start to feel better and then you feel like you are going backwards. Your symptoms may go away or are alleviated, and then all of a sudden they return again. Instead of getting discouraged, try stinging the entry/exit points!

5. Choose a specific point on the L based on the name of the point. This is called treating by the spirit of the point. Look at the names of all the points on the L pathway. Do any of the names jump out at you? What about Greatest Hole (L-6)? Do you ever feel like you are in a very deep hole and you cannot get out? Or how about Narrow Defile (L-7)? Do you ever feel like you barely have room to move? It's like being "between a rock and a hard place?" These are just two examples of some of the points on the L that might speak to you.

6. There is also a Window of the Sky on the L pathway (L-3). This would also be a good spirit point to work out your relationship with you father and your Heavenly Father. This point is forbidden for bee stings, use acupressure only.

7. Try combining any of the above recommendations. "BEE" creative. And remember to keep good records.

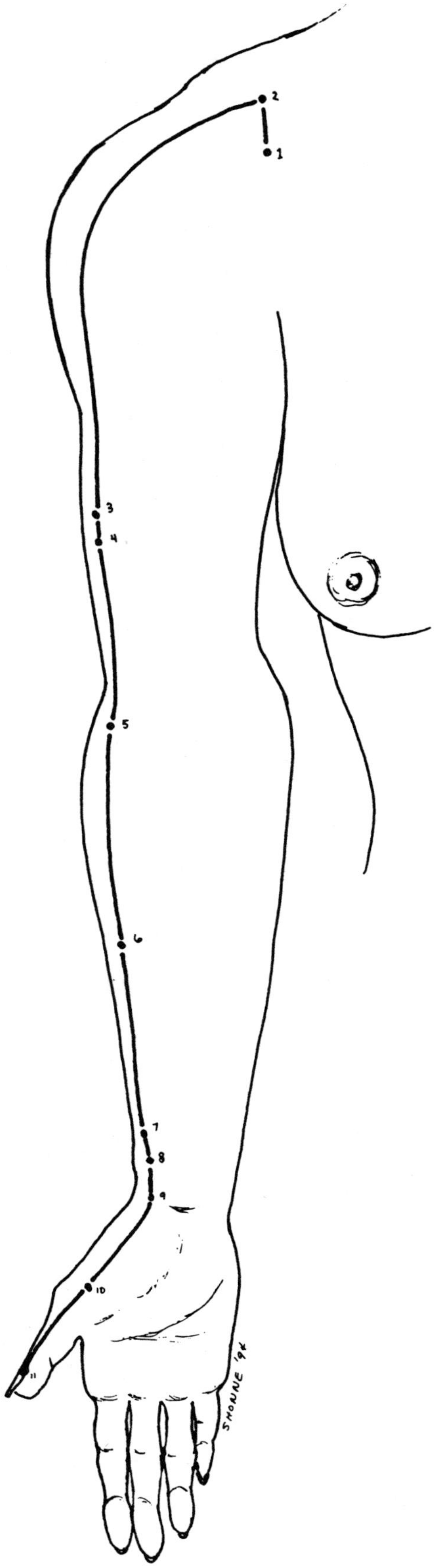

LUNG PATHWAY

LUNG PATHWAY (L)

L-1 Central Treasury (entry pt., first aid pt: drowning)

L-2 Cloud Gate (this is a very spiritual pt.)

F L-3 Celestial Storehouse (Window of the Sky)(use acupressure only)

L-4 Guarding White

L-5 Outside Marsh (water and sedation pts.)

L-6 Greatest Hole (very good pt. for deep depression, fear, tension headaches and elbow trouble)

L-7 Narrow Defile (junction and exit pts. A good spirit pt. if you are stuck "between a rock and a hard place," or are repeating an experience over and over again; good for skin disorders, ice cold limbs and bones.)

L-8 Meridian Gutter (metal, home element, and horary pts., 3 a.m.—5 a.m., first aid pt: electric shock. This is a wonderful pt. in the autumn, especially if the person is dreaming about death or has a fear of dying. This pt. is good when heat and cold are all out of proportion in the hands.)

L-9 Very Great Abyss, the Grand Canyon Pt. (earth, tonification and source pts., first aid pt. for shock and asphyxia, cold hands and feet, can't grasp objects, loss of sensations in fingers, insomnia; facial neuralgia. This is a good spirit pt. for feeling like you are in a deep, dark hole. You can see everyone else up there in the light but you feel like you can't get there.)

L-10 Fish Border (fire pt. This pt. will warm up the metal in the body so it is good for rigidity, good for asthma and hayfever)

L-11 Little Merchant (wood pt. and first aid pt: convulsions, sunstroke, numbness of hands and arms)

The F refers to points which are forbidden to sting.

TREATMENT PLAN FOR THE COLON PATHWAY (CO)

Here is a possible treatment plan to work on the colon (CO) pathway. This plan is immediately followed by point names and locations.

1. If you want to strengthen the CO pathway, you can sting the tonification point (CO-11) or the source point (CO-4).

2. If you want to connect the CO to its paired meridian the lung (L), sting yourself on the junction point (CO-6). (See glossary for more information.)

3. You can enhance the effectiveness of your treatment by stinging the home element point (CO-1). This is best done as a horary treatment, which means a treatment on the home element point at the right time of day (5 a.m.—7 a.m.) and/or in the right season (autumn).

4. If you are having symptoms between 5 a.m.—7 a.m. (i.e., waking up at that time every morning), then you may want to sting the entry point (CO-4) and/or use acupressure on the exit point (CO-20). Another reason to consider entry/exit points is if you start to feel better and then you feel like you are going backwards. Your symptoms may go away or are alleviated, and then all of a sudden they return again. Instead of getting discouraged, try treating the entry/exit points!

5. Choose a specific point on the CO based on the name of the point. This is called treating by the spirit of the point. Look at the names of all the points on the CO pathway. Do any of the names jump out at you? What about "The Great Letting Go," also called Union Valley (CO-4)? Does that sound like you? Do you have trouble letting go of the past? Or what about Shoulder Bone (CO-15)? That might be a good point if you are having shoulder or arm problems. These are just two examples of some of the points on the CO that might speak to you.

6. You could also do a Window to the Sky, Support and Rush Out (CO-18). This will bring the body, mind and spirit together. This is a great spirit point for surrendering to the universe and going with the flow.

7. Try combining any of the above recommendations. "BEE" creative. And remember to keep good records.

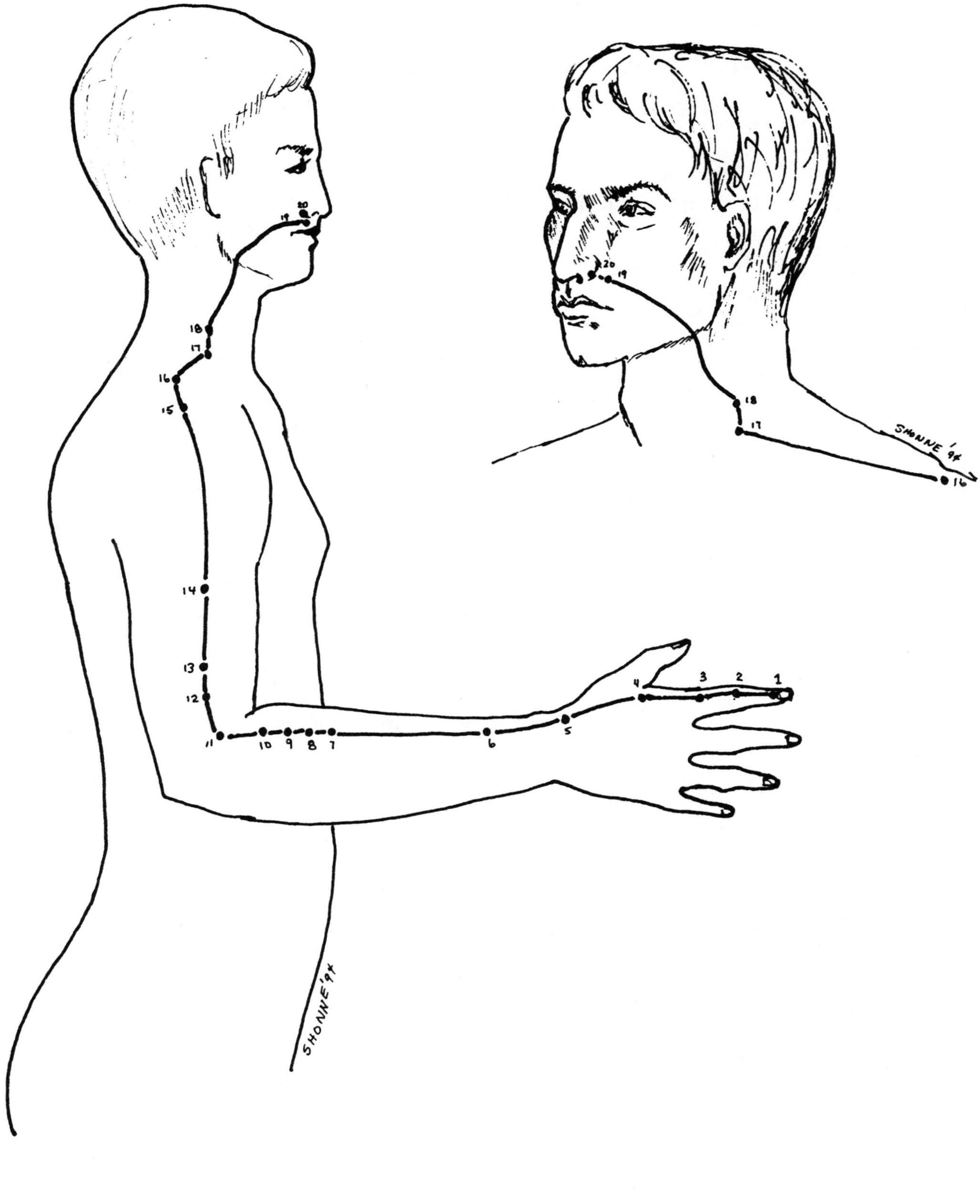

SHONNE '94
SHONNE '94

COLON PATHWAY (CO)

CO-1 Merchant Yang (metal, home element, and horary pts., 5 a.m.—7 a.m., as well as first aid pt: toothache, frozen shoulder, neck problems)

CO-2 Second Space (water and sedation pts., good pt. for rigidity or feeling bone dry, inability to lift arm)

CO-3 Third Space (wood pt.)

CO-4 Union Valley, also known as "The Great Letting Go" (entry and source pts. as well as a center of energy; first aid pt: dull pains, earache, fainting, headaches and spots in front of eyes, food poisoning, poison and toothache. This is an important spirit pt. for letting go of the past!)

CO-5 Yang Stream (fire pt., good pt. for tinnitus, deafness)

CO-6 Side Passage (junction pt.)

CO-7 Warm Flow (good pt. for a patient who feels there's "no good in life," speech difficulties)

CO-8 Lower Ridge (good for headaches, speech problems)

CO-9 Upper Ridge (good for brain fatigue, arthritic knee, paralysis, loss of sensation of limbs)

CO-10 Arm Three Miles (good for rheumatism, arthritis, trouble bending and raising arms, goiters)

CO-11 Pool at the Bend (earth and tonification pts. This is a very good pt. for tennis elbow and arm problems, toothaches, eye problems, pleurisy, asthma, hayfever, bronchitis.)

CO-12 Elbow Bone

CO-13 Arm Five Miles

CO-14 Outer Bone of the Arm

CO-15 Shoulder Bone (first aid pt: shoulder, concussion, electric shock, exhaustion, shock and head injury)

CO-16 Great Bone

CO-17 Celestial Tripod

CO-18 Support and Rush Out (Window of the Sky and a good spirit pt. for surrendering to a Higher Power and letting things go)

F CO-19 Grain Bone-Hole (use acupressure only)

CO-20 Welcome Fragrance (exit pt. and good pt for sinus problems, allergies and clogged nose)

The **F** refers to points which are forbidden to sting.

TREATMENT PLAN FOR THE BLADDER PATHWAY (BL)

Here is a possible treatment plan to work on the bladder (BL) pathway. This plan is immediately followed by point names and locations.

1. If you want to strengthen the BL pathway, you can sting the tonification point (BL-67) or the source point (BL-64). (See glossary for more information.)

2. If you want to connect the BL to its paired meridian the kidney (K), sting yourself on the junction point (BL-58).

3. You can enhance the effectiveness of your treatment by stinging the home element point (BL-66). This is best done as a horary treatment, which means a treatment on the home element point at the right time of day (3 p.m.—5 p.m.) and/or in the right season (winter).

4. If you are having symptoms every day between 3 p.m.—5 p.m. (i.e., a consistent pattern of feeling very tired, like someone just "pulled the plug"), then you may want to use acupressure on the entry point (BL-1), since it is forbidden to sting this point. You can sting the exit point (BL-67). Another reason to consider using the entry/exit points is if you start to feel better and then you feel like you are going backwards. Your symptoms may go away or are alleviated, and then all of a sudden they return again. Instead of getting discouraged, try treating the entry/exit points!

5. Choose a specific point on the BL based on the name of the point. This is called treating by the spirit of the point. Look at the names of all the points on the BL pathway. Do any of the names jump out at you? What about Fly and Scatter (BL-58)? Does that sound like you? Are you feeling scattered and do you need a little peace and quiet? This is just one example of some of the points on the BL that might speak to you.

6. Or how about a Window of the Sky, Celestial Pillar (BL-10)? This point will help to bring the body, mind and spirit together. Even the name of the point makes you think of a heavenly pillar standing straight and tall.

7. Try combining any of the above recommendations. "BEE" creative. And remember to keep good records.

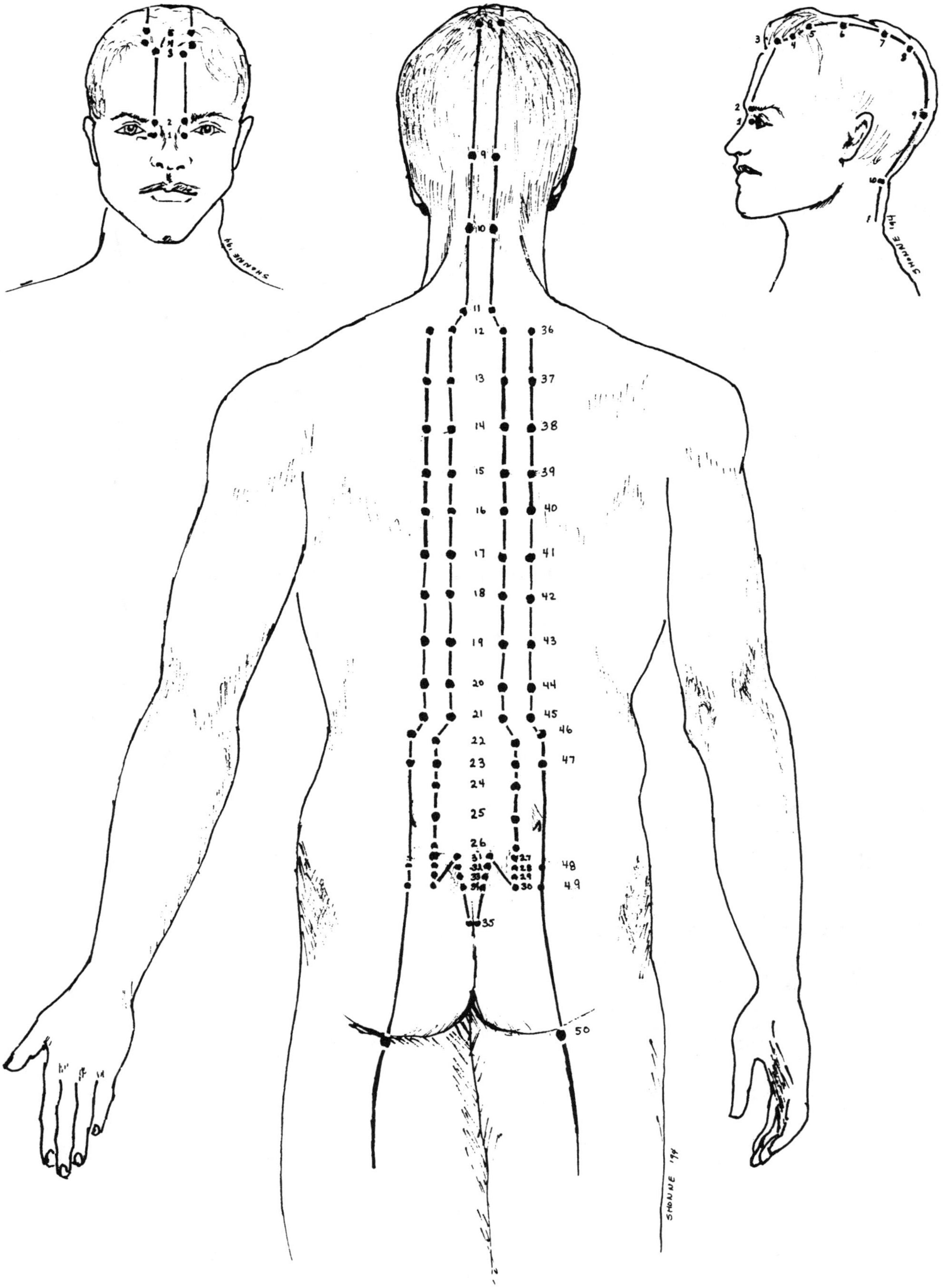

BLADDER PATHWAY

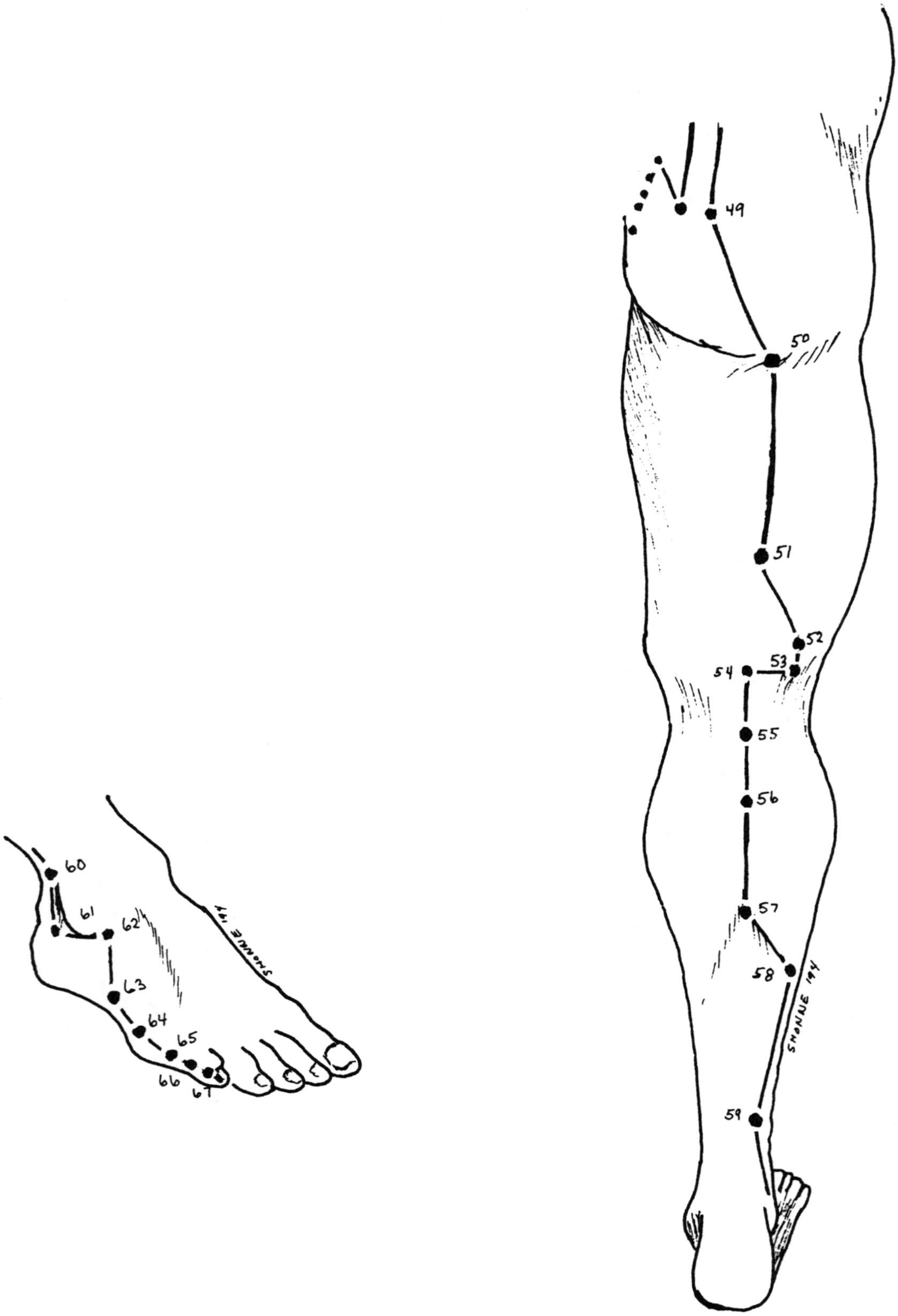

BLADDER PATHWAY

BLADDER PATHWAY (BL)

F BL-1 Bright Eyes (entry pt.)(use acupressure only)

F BL-2 Bamboo Gathering (use acupressure only)

F BL-3 Eyebrows Rushing (use acupressure only)

BL-4 Deviating Turn

BL-5 Five Places

BL-6 Receive Light

BL-7 Celestial Connection

BL-8 Declining Connection Lou End

BL-9 Jade Pillow

BL-10 Celestial Pillar (Window of the Sky)

BL-11 Great Shuttle (External Dragon pt., first aid pt: fractures and sprains)

BL-12 Wind Gate

BL-13 Lung Shu

BL-14 Heart Protector Shu

BL-15 Heart Shu

BL-16 Governor Shu

BL-17 Diaphragm Shu

The F refers to points which are forbidden to sting.

BL-18 Liver Shu

BL-19 Gall Bladder Shu

BL-20 Spleen Shu

BL-21 Stomach Shu

BL-22 Three Heater Shu

BL-23 Kidney Shu

BL-24 Sea of *Ch'i* Shu

BL-25 Colon Shu

BL-26 First Gate Shu

BL-27 Small Intestine Shu

BL-28 Bladder Shu

BL-29 Central Backbone Shu

BL-30 White Ring Shu

BL-31 Upper Bone-Hole

BL-32 Second Bone-Hole

BL-33 Central Bone-Hole

BL-34 Lower Bone-Hole

BL-35 Meeting of Yang

BL-36 Near Division

BL-37 Soul Door, or Gate of Abundance (spirit pt. for the Lungs)

BL-38 Superficial Cleft, also known as The Happy Point (spirit pt. for Heart Protector)

BL-39 Bend Yang (spirit pt. for the Heart)

BL-40 Wail of Grief

BL-41 Diaphragm Border

BL-42 Spiritual Soul Gate (spirit pt. for the Liver)

BL-43 Yang Net (spirit pt. for the Gall Bladder)

BL-44 Thought Dwelling (spirit pt. for the Spleen)

BL-45 Stomach Granary (spirit pt. for the Stomach)

BL-46 Diaphragm Gate of Vitality (spirit pt. for the Three Heater)

BL-47 Ambition Room (spirit pt. for the Kidneys)

BL-48 Womb and Heart Diaphragm (spirit pt. for the Bladder)

BL-49 Orderly Frontier

BL-50 Receive and Support (good first aid pt. for muscles)

BL-51 Prosperous Gate

BL-52 Floating Reserve

BL-53 Equilibrium Yang

BL-54 Equilibrium Middle (earth pt., first aid pt: spinal injury, skin diseases, arthritis of knee, night sweats and stiff neck)

BL-55 Uniting Yang

BL-56 Supporting Muscles

BL-57 Supporting Mountain

BL-58 Fly and Scatter, Taking Flight (junction pt., good pt. to calm down; center of energy pt., good first aid pt. for strengthening vitality, also good for weakness of legs, cystitis, constipation, and lumbago)

BL-59 Instep Yang (first aid pt: food poisoning, elimination of toxins, both physical and mental)

BL-60 Kunlun Mountains (fire pt., first aid pt: anxiety, facial neuralgia, fractures, spinal injury, sprains; inability to do things, can't turn neck and elbow, swelling of feet and hands, glandular disease, sciatica. This pt. is good for fear in relationships.)

BL-61 Servant's Aide (External Dragon's pt., first aid pt. for pain in knee, spasm in calf, can't raise the knee, needs help up stairs and getting in car)

BL-62 Extended Meridian (good pt. for diseases of the spine)

BL-63 Metal Gate (good pt. for swelling, tinnitus)

BL-64 Capital Bone (source pt., first aid pt: bee stings, stiff neck, lumbago, red eyes)

BL-65 Bone Binder (wood, sedation pts., first aid pt: burns, cystitis, food poisoning, insect bites, poison, scalds, sunburn, urine retention and frequency, difficulty healing a bone, fear of wind and cold, sciatica)

BL-66 Penetrating Valley (water, home element, and horary pts., 3 p.m.-5 p.m., good pt. for blurred vision, dreams of drowning and falling, fear of the unknown, worrying about "What's going to happen next?," stiffness in neck, pain in feet and calves, edema)

BL-67 Reaching Yin (metal, tonification, and exit pts.)

TREATMENT PLAN FOR THE KIDNEY PATHWAY (K)

Here is a possible treatment plan to work on the kidney (K) pathway. This plan is immediately followed by point names and locations.

1. If you want to strengthen the K pathway, you can sting the tonification point (K-7) or the source point (K-3).

2. If you want to connect the K to its paired meridian the bladder (BL), sting yourself on the junction point (K-4). (See glossary for more information.)

3. You can enhance the effectiveness of your treatment by stinging the home element point (K-10). This is best done as a horary treatment, which means a treatment on the home element point at the right time of day (5 p.m.— 7 p.m.) and/or in the right season (winter).

4. If you are having symptoms every day between 5 p.m.—7 p.m. (i.e., feeling very tired or feeling like someone has "just pulled the plug"), then you may want to sting the entry point (K-1) and/or the exit point (K-22). If you have trouble finding this point on a woman you can also use K-27. Another reason to consider stinging the entry/exit points is if you start to feel better and then you feel like you are going backwards. Your symptoms may go away or are alleviated, and then all of a sudden they return again. Instead of getting discouraged, try stinging the entry/exit points!

5. Choose a specific point on the K based on the name of the point. This is called treating by the spirit of the point. Look at the names of all the points on the K pathway. Do any of the names jump out at you? What about Spirit Burial Ground (K-24)? This is a wonderful point for resurrecting the spirit in someone after they feel that a part of them has died. Does that sound like you? Or how about Shining Sea (K-6)? This is like looking in a pond of water, seeing your reflection, and gaining insight from what you see. These are just two examples of some of the points on the K that might speak to you.

6. Try combining any of the above recommendations. "BEE" creative. And remember to keep good records.

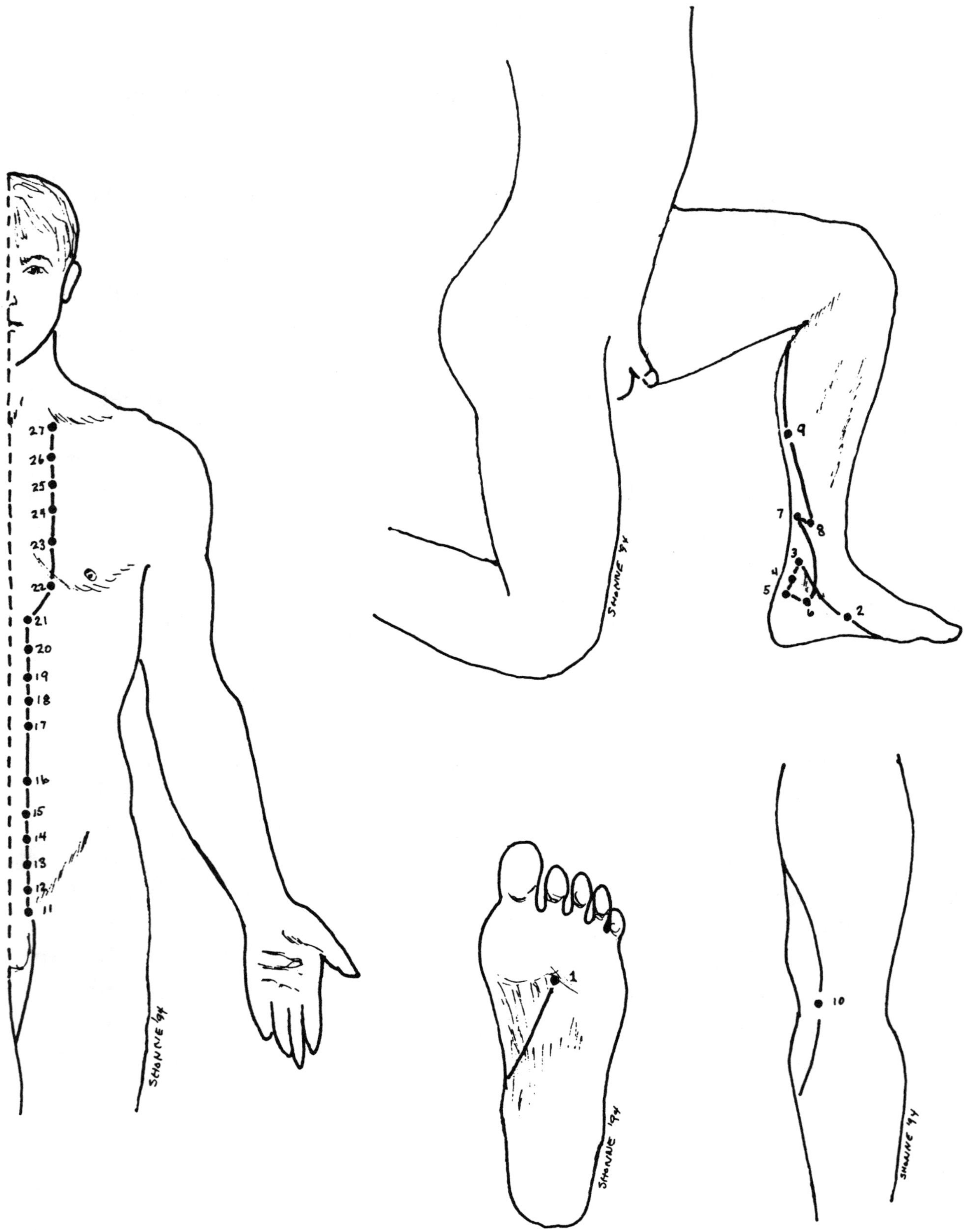

KIDNEY PATHWAY

KIDNEY PATHWAY (K)

K-1 Gushing Spring (wood, sedation, and entry pts., first aid pt: retention of fluid and beet red face)

K-2 Blazing Valley (fire pt., first aid pt: cystitis, night sweats and impotence)

K-3 Greater Mountain Stream (earth and source pts., first aid pt: dryness, sore throat, insomnia, migraines, epilepsy, irregular menses, limbs weary and heavy)

K-4 Large Goblet (junction pt., first aid pt: blurred vision, depression before period)

K-5 Water Spring (first aid pt: problems with base of the spine, fear and depression together, agoraphobia)

K-6 Shining Sea (first aid pt: bee stings, concussion, very dark urine and pains in chest; a good spirit pt. for illumination)

K-7 Recover Flow (metal and tonification pts., lots of sweating or none at all)

K-8 Exchange Pledges (menstrual disorders, uterus prolapse)

K-9 Guest House (weakness in legs, spasms, twitches)

K-10 Yin Valley (water, home element, and horary pts., 5 p.m.—7 p.m. first aid pt: excessive perspiration, vaginal discharge, depression, watering eyes, pain around genitals, swollen painful abdomen)

K-11 Pubic Bone

K-12 Great Brightness

K-13 Door of Infants (center of energy pt.)

K-14 Four Full

K-15 Middle Flowing Out

K-16 Vitals Correspondence

K-17 Merchant Crooked

K-18 Stone Pass

K-19 Yin Capital

K-20 Open Valley

K-21 Dark Gate

K-22 Walking on the Veranda (exit pt.; picture yourself walking on a veranda)

K-23 Spirit Seal (first aid pt: sunstroke. This is a spirit pt. to help you remember who you really are and what you came here to do.)

K-24 Spirit Burial Ground, Spirit Ruins (a great pt. to resurrect the spirit, after a part of you has died)

K-25 Spirit Storehouse

K-26 Amidst Elegance

K-27 Storehouse

CHAPTER 8

TREATMENT PLAN FOR THE CONCEPTION VESSEL (CV)

This pathway is not ruled by the five elements. The conception vessel is part of the 8 extra meridians. Here are some possible reasons why you might want to use the CV:

1. This pathway is the most yin pathway in the body. Go to this pathway if you need to go inward, go home. This pathway will bring someone into themselves.

2. Go to this pathway if you are doing pretty well but just need a little push in the right direction.

The CV points are named on page 158-159 and shown on page 157. Here are some possible points you can use on the conception vessel:

1. If some one has a cold lower abdomen and/or is trying to get pregnant, this is a good point (CV-4), First Gate.

2. CV-3 (Central Pole) is a good point for the bladder and a center of energy.

3. CV-6 (Sea of *Ch'i*) is a good point to bring nourishment.

4. CV-8 (Spirit Tower Gate) is a wonderful point to build up someone's spirit. May relate to birth trauma. This is the umbilicus, so take care here. I wouldn't do this pt. very early in treatment due to possible swelling.

5. If you have had a severe blow to the top of the head or the very base of the spine, you may want to do the entry/exit points for CV and GV with acupressure or perhaps bee stings (CV-1, CV-24; GV-1, GV-28).

6. Choose a specific point on the pathway based on the name of the point. This is called treating by the spirit of the point. Look at all the names of points on the list for the CV. Do any of those names jump out at you? For example,

what about Stone Gate (CV-5)? Do you sometimes feel like you are banging your head against a wall? Is there a stone in the way that prevents you from getting out of the gate? Then you may want to consider Stone Gate. What about Chest Center (CV-17)? Do you carry everything within? Does this sound like you? These are just two examples of some of the points on the CV that might speak to you.

7. Consider going to a Window of the Sky, Celestial Chimney (CV-22). Remember that Windows bring the body, mind and spirit together. This is a very helpful point for people who have trouble receiving love and compassion. If you don't want to do a bee sting on this point, you can use gentle pressure.

8. Try combining any of the above recommendations. "BEE" creative. And remember to keep good records.

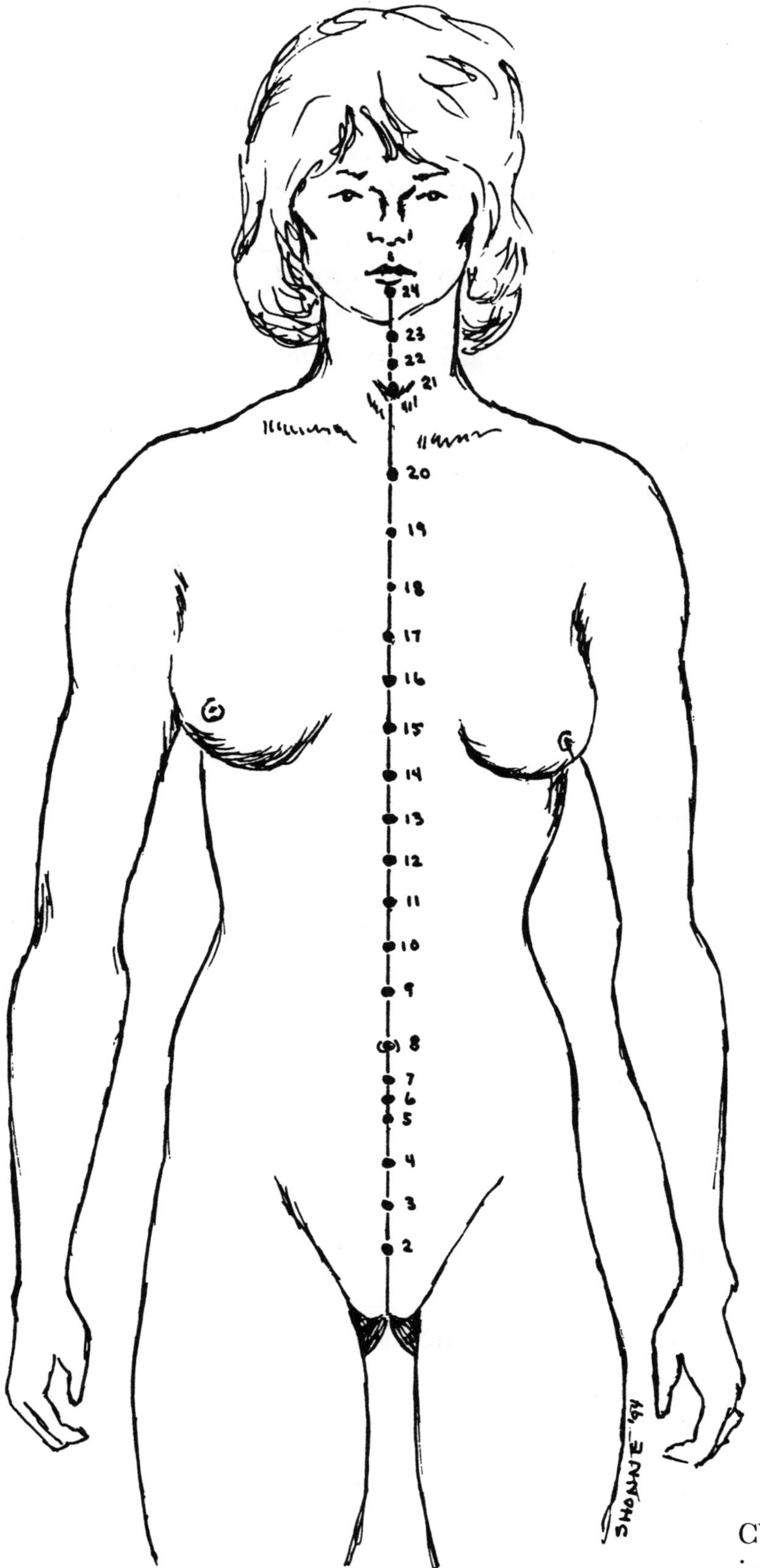

CV-1 is located
in the perineum

CONCEPTION VESSEL (CV)

CV-1 Meeting of Yin (entry pt. and first aid pt: drowning. This is a spirit pt. for feeling like you're drowning in a sea of emotions. This point is located in the perineum; you may want to use only acupressure.)

CV-2 Curved Bone (good for impotency)

CV-3 Central Pole (center of energy and first aid pt: urinary problems)

F CV-4 Origin Pass (center of energy and this pt. can affect the small intestine, also good for infertility; forbidden during pregnancy)

F CV-5 Stone Gate (main center of energy, a pt. related to the three heater pathway and body temperature, good for infertility; forbidden in pregnancy)

CV-6 Sea of *Ch'i* (main center of energy)

CV-7 Yin Intersection (affects warmth in the lower abdomen, good for infertility and menstrual disorders)

CV-8 Spirit Tower Gate (great spirit pt. for birth trauma and loneliness)

CV-9 Water Divide

F CV-10 Lower Venter (forbidden in pregnancy)

CV-11 Interior Strengthening (good for edema)

CV-12 Middle Venter (center of energy)

CV-13 Upper Venter

CV-14 Great Tower Gate (affects the heart and first aid for sea and travel sickness)

The **F** refers to points which are forbidden to sting.

CV-15 Turtledove Tail (Internal Dragon pt. and an alarm pt. for the heart protector)

CV-16 Central Palace

CV-17 Chest Center (sea of energy and a pt. affecting breathing)

CV-18 Jade Hall

CV-19 Purple Palace

CV-20 Flower Covering

CV-21 Jade Pivot

CV-22 Celestial Chimney (Window of the Sky, a spirit pt. for those who have trouble receiving love and support)(You can use gentle pressure here if you don't want to do a bee sting.)

F CV-23 Ridge Spring (you can use gentle acupressure)

CV-24 Receiving Fluid (exit pt.)

The **F** refers to points which are forbidden to sting.

TREATMENT PLAN FOR THE GOVERNOR VESSEL (GV)

The Governor Vessel (GV) is not ruled by the five elements. It is part of the 8 extra meridians. The GV points are named on page 163-164 and shown on page 162. Here are some possible reasons why you might want to go to the GV:

1. It is the most predominantly yang pathway in the body. It is like sunlight and connects you with the heavens. It is outwardly moving and is filled with powerful energy.

2. This pathway will tend to bring someone outside of themselves.

3. This is a good pathway to go to if you are doing pretty well, but you need a little push in the right direction, in this case out into the world.

Here are some possible points you can use on the Governor Vessel:

1. A good first aid point concussions, fractures and spinal injuries is Lumbar Yang Pass (GV-3)

2. Contracted Muscle (GV-8) is good for tight muscles.

3. Meeting of 100 Ancestors (GV-20) is a very good point for epilepsy and just calming the spirit in general.

4. If you've had a severe blow to the top of the head or the very base of the spine, you can use acupressure or bee stings on the entry/exit points on CV and GV.

5. Choose a specific point on the GV based on the name of the point. This is called treating by the spirit of the point. Look at the names of all the points on the GV. Do any of the names jump out at you? What about Gate of Life (GV-4)? This is for people who are not open to life. This point gives them a little push outward. (GV-4 is forbidden to sting for people under the age of 20.) Are you feeling depressed or hopeless? Do you feel like nothing is ever going to change. Consider this point: It will push you into your destiny. Now, look at Body Pillar (GV-12). Go to this point when there is no backbone on the body, mind, spirit

level. You might feel like you're "crumbling." This point is very good for someone who gets sick a lot and has no center. It is also helpful for someone who is too rigid. And don't forget about GV-14, Great Hammer! This is a great point for hitting someone over the head and pushing them in the direction they are already going. These are just three examples of some of the points on the GV that might speak to you.

6. You might also want to consider a Window of the Sky, Wind Mansion (GV-16). Keep in mind that Windows bring the body, mind and spirit together. This point will bring you closer to the heavens if you are shut down (if your Window is closed) or it can close your Window if it is too open (you are not grounded). This point is forbidden to bee sting, but you can use acupressure instead.

7. Try combining any of the above recommendations. "BEE" creative. And remember to keep good records.

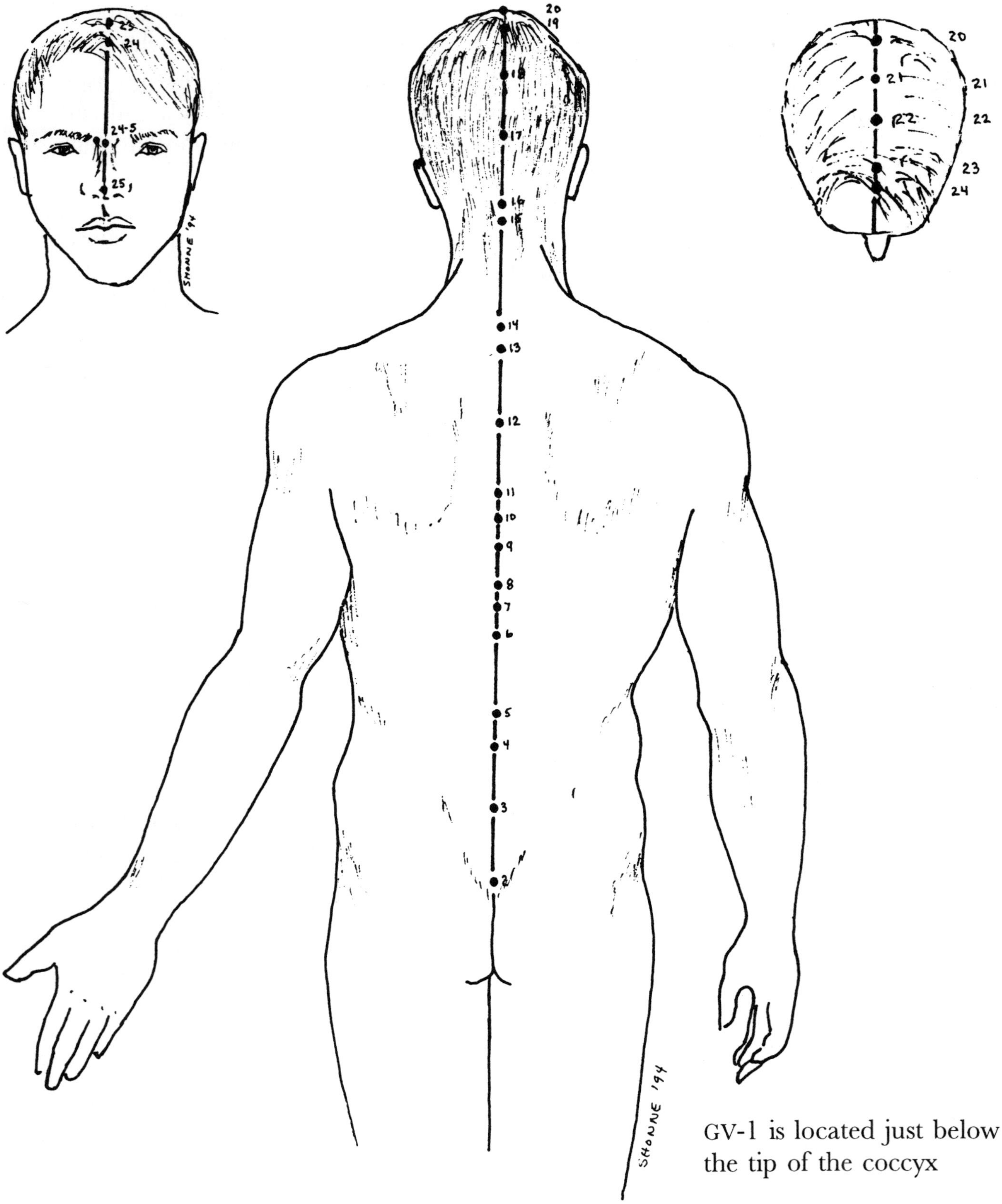

GV-1 is located just below the tip of the coccyx

GOVERNOR VESSEL (GV)

GV-1 Long Strong (entry pt. This point is located just below the coccyx; you may want to use only acupressure.)

GV-2 Lumbar Shu

GV-3 Lumbar Yang Pass (first aid pt: concussion, fractures, sprains and spinal injury)

F GV-4 Gate of Life (spirit pt. to bring someone back to life; forbidden under the age of 20)

GV-5 Suspended Pivot (good pt. for rigidity and stiffness)

F GV-6 Middle of the Spine (you can use acupressure)

GV-7 Central Pivot

GV-8 Contracted Muscle (this is a good pt. for muscle spasms)

GV-9 Utmost Yang

GV-10 Spirit Tower

GV-11 Spirit Path

GV-12 Body Pillar (a good pt. for strength and standing straight, good for rheumatic diseases)

GV-13 Kiln Path (good for rigid shoulders)

GV-14 Great Hammer (reunion pt. for the following pathways: SI, BL, TH, GB, CO, ST and GV. Also a first aid pt. for colds. This is a spirit pt. when someone needs to be hit over the head with a hammer to get them moving in the right direction. It is also helpful if you thought you were

---

The **F** refers to points which are forbidden to sting.

over an emotional problem and it keeps coming back. This pt. is also good for stiff necks.)

F GV-15 Mute's Gate (sea of bone marrow and a good pt. for muteness) (use acupressure only)

F GV-16 Wind Mansion (Window of the Sky, sea of bone marrow)(use acupressure only)

F GV-17 Brain Door (use acupressure only)

GV-18 Strength Divider

GV-19 Posterior Summit (sea of bone marrow)

GV-20 Ancestors of 100 Meetings (sea of bone marrow, External Dragon pt. and good pt. for epilepsy and to calm the spirit)

GV-21 Anterior Summit

GV-22 Skull Meeting

GV-23 Upper Star

GV-24 Spirit Hall

GV-24.5 This pt. has no name but it is approximately in the location of the third eye.

F GV-25 White Bone Hole (use acupressure only)

GV-26 Middle of Man

F GV-27 Correct Exchange (use acupressure only)

GV-28 Mouth Crossing (I recommend using acupressure only)

The **F** refers to points which are forbidden to sting.

SPECIAL POINTS

The following points are considered special points that have been used for common ailments over the years. You may want to explore these along with the other points you are using. These points were gleaned from a variety of sources that are listed in the Reading List.

These may be used as points to treat chronic conditions or first aid points for acute conditions. Remember, if you sting the extremities (arms and legs) within the first month of treatment you may have a great deal of swelling. Please do not use this chapter without reading the sections on "Reactions" and "Warnings." I recommend that if you want to use these points, you do so in conjunction with the Five element points.

ALLERGIES: LV-3, CO-4 & 11, TH-5, BL-10, K-27, CV-6, ST-36

ANEMIA: BL-38

ANKLE PROBLEMS: K-3 & 6, BL-60 & 62, GB-40

ASTHMA: GV-10, HP-8, L-10

ANXIETY: BL-10, TH-15, CV-17, HP-3 & 6, H-7

ARM PROBLEMS: TH-9,14, & 15, GB-20 & 21

ARTHRITIS: CO-4 & 11, TH-5 & 6, ST-36 & 39, GB-20
OF THE KNEE: BL-54 & 55

BACK PAIN: BL-23, 25, 47, 48, 50, 51 & 54, CV-6, SP-8

BALANCE: TH-3

BELL'S PALSY: SI-5

BLADDER PROBLEMS: BL-58 & 65, LV-8 , K-2

BLURRED VISION: BL-66, K-4, LV-3

BONE MARROW PROBLEMS: GB-39

COLDS/FLU: GB-20, K-27, CO-4, BL-10, CV-22

COLD LIMBS: ST-37, SP-2

CONSTIPATION: CV-6, ST-36, CO-4 & 11, BL-25 & 28

CO-ORDINATION PROBLEMS: TH-8, GB-34, 37 & 40

CORTISONE PRODUCTION: GB-39

COUGHS: ST-43, L-7 & 9

CHRONIC FATIGUE: L-1, GB-20 & 21, TH-2, 3, 5, 14, & 15, HP-6, ST-36, BL-23 & 47, CV-6, LV-3, SP-5 & 6, CO-15 & 16, SI-10, 12, 13, & 14

CRAMPS, SPASMS: BL-52, 53, 56 & 57, LV-3 & 4, K-9, GB-34 & 37

DEPRESSION : TH-5, CV-17, L-1, K-27, BL-1O, 23, 38 & 47, GV-19, 20 & 21, GB-20, CO-7, HP-6, ST-9 & 10

DEPRESSION BEFORE PERIOD: K-4

DIARRHEA: ST-36, LV-2, CV-6, SP-4

DIZZINESS: TH-3

EAR PROBLEMS: K-3, TH-2

ELBOW PROBLEMS: L-6, CO-11

EPILEPSY: GV-9, HP-9, ST-36 & 41, SI-3, TH-8

EYE PROBLEMS: GV-14, GB-1 (with care), 37 & 20, CO-4

BLURRED VISION: BL-66, LV-3, K-4

FINGER PROBLEMS: TH-4, L-9

FRUSTRATION: GB-20, 21 & 30, BL-48, L-1, CV-17, CV -12

GOITER: GB-38, CO-10

GOUT: ST-41

HANDS (HARD TO GRASP THINGS): TH-4, L-9 , SI-9

HAIR (FALLING OUT): ST-39

HIP: GB-28, 29 & 30
IF YOU HAVE A HIP PROBLEM ON ONE SIDE DO CO-18 ON THE OTHER SIDE OF THE BODY

HEADACHES: GB-20 & 41, BL-10, CO-4, LV-3
FOR HEADACHES AT THE TOP OF THE HEAD: BL-6 & 7

HOT FLASHES: K-1 & 2, GB-2, CO-4, K-27, CV-17, GV-20

IMMUNE SYSTEM: K-3 & 27, CV-6 & 17, ST-36, LV-3, BL-23, 36 THROUGH 40, & 47, CO-11, TH-5 & 14, SI-14

INSOMNIA: SP-6, GB-2, BL-10, 38, 61 & 62, H-7, HP-6, CV-17, K-6 & 25, L-9

KNEE PROBLEMS: CO-9, ST-35 & 36, GB-34 & 44, LV-7 & 8, K-10, SP-9, BL-53, 54 & 61

MEMORY/CONCENTRATION: GV-20, GB-20, BL-10, CV-17, ST-36, LV-3

MIGRAINES: K-3, LV-3

NECK PAIN: GV-16, GB-20 & 21, TH-15 & 16, BL-6, 12 & 20

NECK, STIFF: SI-3, 16 & 17, BL-10, 54, 60, 64, 66, ST-6, GV-19

NIGHT SWEATS: BL -54, K-2

NUMBNESS (GENERAL): SP-6 & 9, TH-1
HANDS & ARMS: L-11
LEGS: CO-9

PAIN (UPPER BODY): GB-20, CO-4

PAIN (LOWER BODY): ST-36, K-3, GB-20, BL-60

PARALYSIS: GB-37, ST-40, GV-2

PMS/CRAMPS: SP-4, 6, 12 & 13, BL-27 THROUGH 34 & 48, CV-4 & 6

RHEUMATISM (NECK & SHOULDERS): BL-8, GB-41

RIGIDITY: CO-2, GV-5 & 12

SCIATICA: BL-10, 23, 47, 48, 50, 54, 60 & 65, CV-6, GB-20, 30 & 40

SKIN DISORDERS: BL-10, 23 & 47, ST-36 & 44, L-10

SHOULDER, FROZEN: TH-1 & 4, CO-1 & 2, GV-13, & ALSO TREAT BL-62 ON THE OPPOSITE SHOULDER.

SHOULDER PAIN: GB-20 & 21, TH-14, 15 & 16, L-6, CO-15 &16, BL-36, SI-10 THROUGH 14

SPASMS: LV-6, GB-34 & 37, LV-3

SPEECH: GB-44, CO-8, ST-40

SPINE PROBLEMS: BL-62, K-5, GV-1 THROUGH 15

TINNITUS: BL-63, CO-5, ST-36, SI-2, 4, & 5

VERTIGO: SI-7

WEAKNESS: BL-58, K-9, LV-6, ST-38

WRIST PAIN: TH-4, TH-5, HP-7, HP-6

CHAPTER 9
MAJOR BLOCKS

If you feel "stuck" or that you've hit a plateau, you may have a major block. It may be time to consider correcting this block. A major block is like a garden hose that is all twisted or has knots in it. You may have to unravel these knots to have a breakthrough.

There are several major blocks you can look into. It is best if they can be corrected by acupuncture needles. If your insurance does not cover acupuncture, you cannot afford it on your own, or if there is no acupuncturist in your area, you can consider stinging yourself on the recommended acupuncture points.

These treatments should be used after the swelling and itching reactions subside—this is usually after the first month or so. These treatments assist the healing process by either cleansing stagnant energy or by correcting chronic blockages in the flow of *Ch'i*. In most of these treatments, you sting all of the indicated points in one session. Generally, you may want to limit your treatments to one of these blocks at a time. The points listed as Windows and Entry/Exit blocks can be done as needed; you may want to add one or two of these points as part of a treatment plan derived from the five element work.

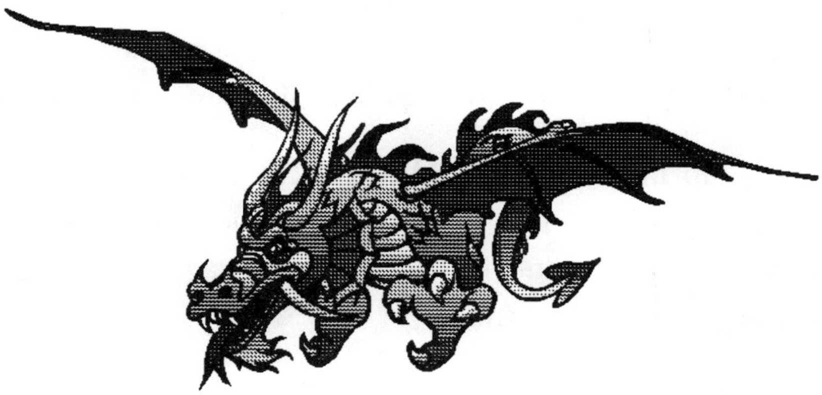

Dragons bring good luck in Chinese philosophy!

THE INTERNAL DRAGONS

This treatment is needed for one who feels stuck in an emotion: anger, joy, worry, grief, or anxiety (fear). It is called the Internal Dragons because it feels like something is coming at you from the inside. This is predominantly an emotional treatment and is therefore very good for depression. Dragons bring good luck in Oriental medicine.

This condition may come from a trauma or an ongoing emotional situation. Here are four indications to signal whether the Internal Dragons are present (usually all indications are present but not always):

1. The person may feel possessed on the inside by something outside of himself, in this case an illness.

2. The patient has trouble making eye contact. He doesn't look you in the eye. You may have the feeling that he is avoiding looking at you in general. You will feel like you are having trouble connecting with this person. He seems distant and far away. It may feel like "nobody's home."

3. The person's life may seem very chaotic.

4. His symptoms have been persistent over a long period of time.

Statements that go with the Internal Dragons may sound similar to these:

- "I have a rip in my soul that I just can't get around."
- "This isn't me. I feel like something else has taken over."
- "I'm feeling out of control; I feel like the rage (worry, grief) has taken over and is controlling me."

To release the 7 Internal Dragons you need the following points:

The master point below CV-15
Stomach-25 (bilaterally)
Stomach-32 (bilaterally)
Stomach-41 (bilaterally)

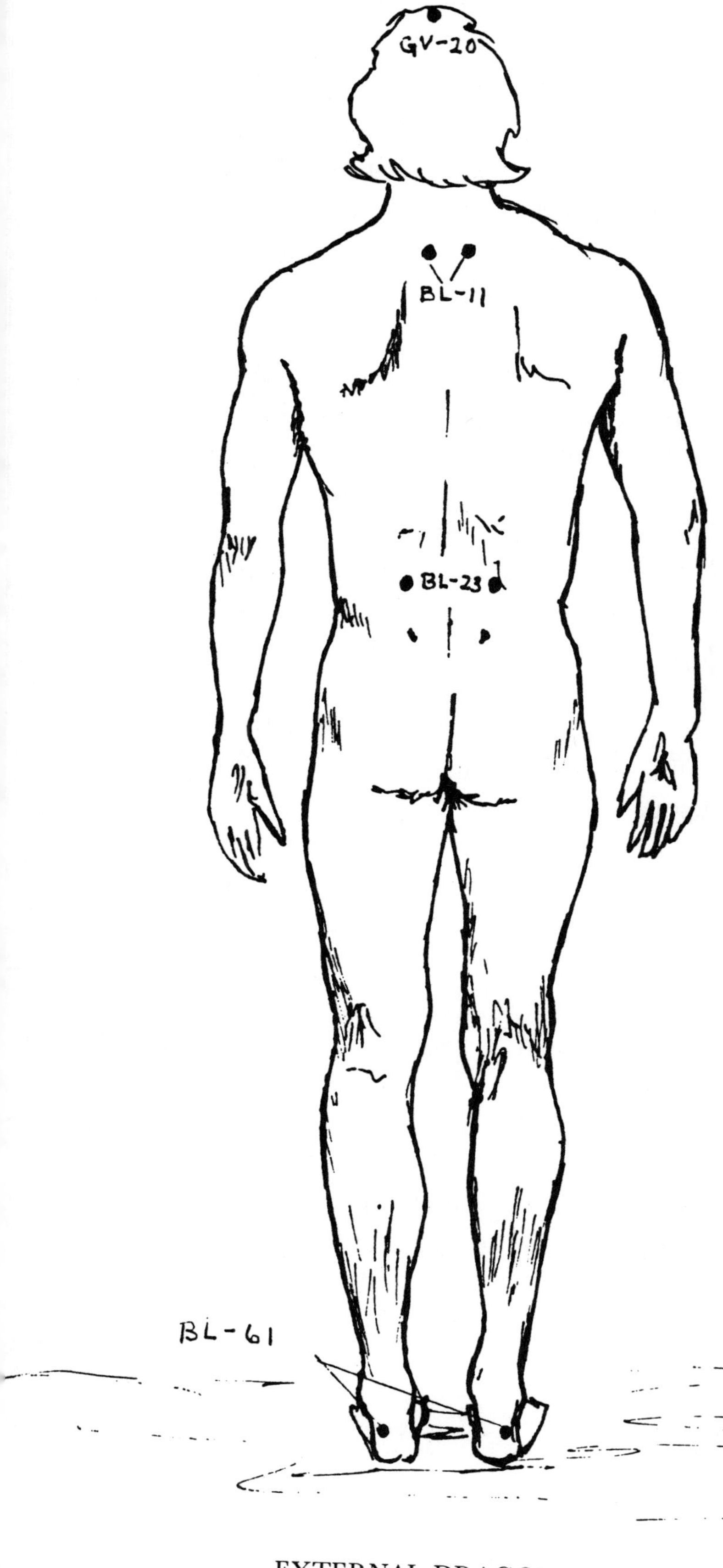

EXTERNAL DRAGONS

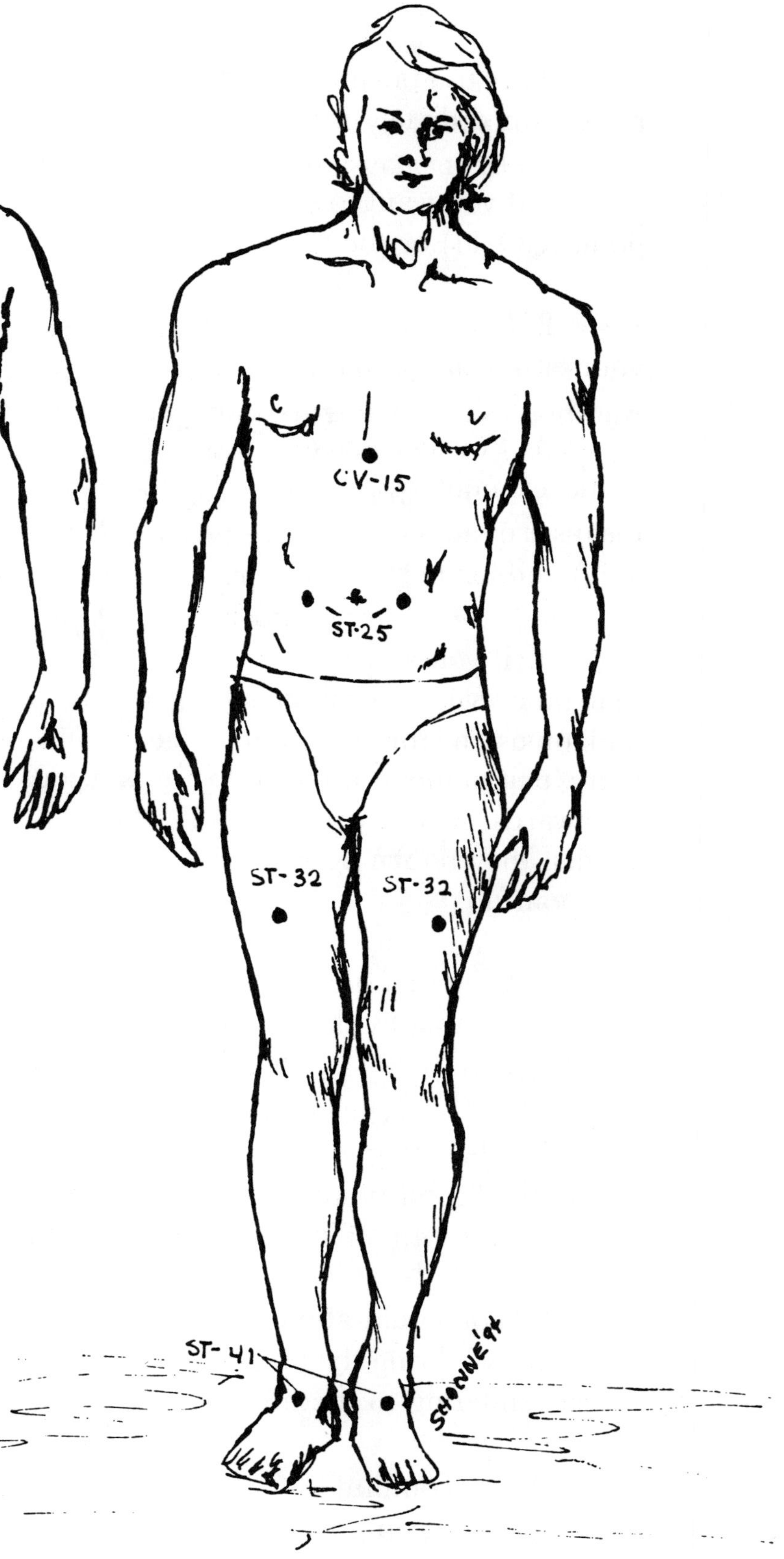

INTERNAL DRAGONS

THE EXTERNAL DRAGONS

This treatment is needed if something came at you from the outside. It could be a disease, a car accident, a rape, a fall, or a major trauma of some kind. This condition may also be present if you were exposed to "the elements" for a period of time, for example: dampness, humidity, fire, heat, cold, wind, or dryness.

Let's say you were outside on a very cold day and ever since then you have not been able to get warm. An extreme example of that would be frostbite. Another example might be if your house caught on fire and you just barely escaped. In this case, you would be exposed to the external fire and heat and perhaps even wind. This would be a perfect example of how the Internal and External Dragons might be needed. If you narrowly escaped from a fire, there would probably be a lot of fear associated with that experience. Then you would treat both the Internal and External Dragons.

The same four indications may be present as listed above for the Internal Dragons, with the main difference being that the person feels very strongly that something came at them from the outside.

Here are the points needed to release the 7 External Dragons and correct the situation:

GV-20
Bladder 11 (bilaterally)
Bladder 23 (bilaterally)
Bladder 61 (bilaterally)

If the person regains good eye contact, then you know the pattern has been broken. I wish you good luck. It is harder to get results if this condition persists. Please keep me posted on your results.

AGGRESSIVE ENERGY (AE)

If left uncontrolled long enough, the K'o cycle will become self-destructive. We call this condition "aggressive energy." When this situation arises, the patient is likely to show some self-destructive behaviors (like drug abuse, car accidents, suicide attempts, etc.) She may also be prone to have illnesses where the body attacks itself, such as cancer, MS, lupus and diseases which are thought to be auto-immune in nature. Aggressive Energy can be drained fairly easily with acupuncture needles.

Aggressive Energy is an invasive energy that knocks us off balance. It is harmful energy that is aimed at controlling the grandson instead of feeding the son. Looking at the chart of the five elements, you can note that the K'o cycle reaches across along the path of the star, rather than around the circle, which is the path of the Shen cycle. It is energy that stagnates and then aggressively moves across the K'o cycle; a metaphor for this would be that the grandmother is sick and turns on the grandchild. AE is a step beyond reasonable control. It is very destructive and deep seated. The danger is to the yin organs: the liver, the heart, the heart protector, the spleen, the lungs and the kidneys. AE can be triggered by an acute or devastating trauma or a chronic condition, i.e., pain or illness.

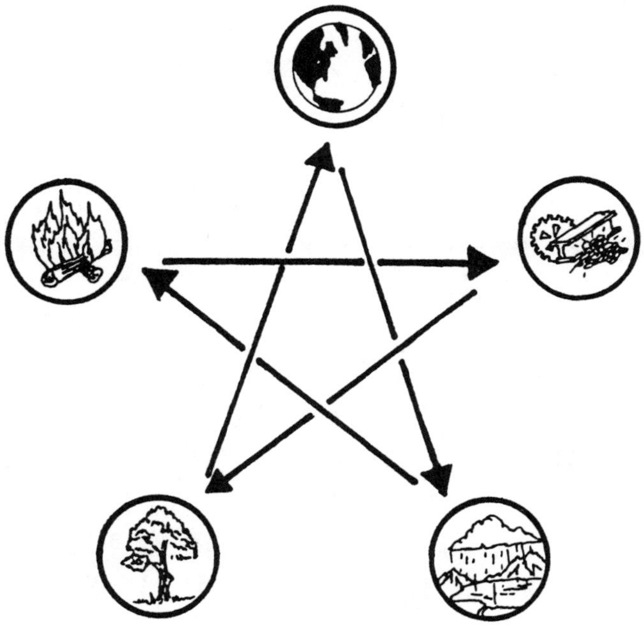

***K'o Cycle:** Aggressive energy moves across the K'o cycle, which occurs when the grandmother is out of balance and the cycle of control becomes destructive.*

So if you have symptoms in a pair of elements which are connected as grandmother—grandchild, then you may Aggressive Energy. For example, if you have troubles in the wood element (for eg., menstrual cramps, problems with tendons and ligaments, one-sided headaches, trouble making decisions) and you also have symptoms in the earth element (for eg., craving sweets, stomach or digestion issues, food allergies, leg and feet problems, feeling misunderstood) then you may have Aggressive Energy.

Another indication that you may have Aggressive Energy is having a chronic illness, especially one thought to be an auto-immune disease, like Cancer, MS, Lupus, AIDS, etc.

A third indication for Aggressive Energy is that you've had a major trauma.

If you have Aggressive Energy you are hard to be around. You are really struggling. You may also be self-absorbed or have some self-destructive behaviors: car accidents, addictions, destructive relationships that you stay stuck in, to name a few.

Also, if you are having a poor response to Bee Venom Therapy, then you may have Aggressive Energy.

OK, so now you think you have Aggressive Energy . . . what do you do now? An acupuncturist can drain this for you. You may want to consider this; it is a very simple procedure. Basically, 12 needles are inserted (very superficially) in the back Shu points for the yin organs. (Three test needles are also used for placebos, or control needles in non-points.) Here is a list of the points that are used. All points are done bilaterally:

BLADDER-13 (FOR THE LUNGS)
BLADDER-14 (FOR THE HEART PROTECTOR)
BLADDER-15 (FOR THE HEART)
BLADDER-18 (FOR THE LIVER)
BLADDER-20 (FOR THE SPLEEN)
BLADDER-23 (FOR THE KIDNEYS)

The acupuncturist should put the needles in very superficially, with no manipulation. If you have AE, a redness will develop around the needle. Sometimes there will be no redness but the person will still benefit from the treatment. What the acupuncturist is doing is draining the harmful energy out of the organs where it has gotten stuck. I like to look at it this way: think of a teapot that is on the stove. The burner is on and the water in the teapot is now boiling. But unfortunately, the hole in the teapot is plugged up and there is no place for the steam to escape. What we are doing, by draining the AE, is making a hole is the teapot for the steam to escape so it doesn't stay so bottled up.

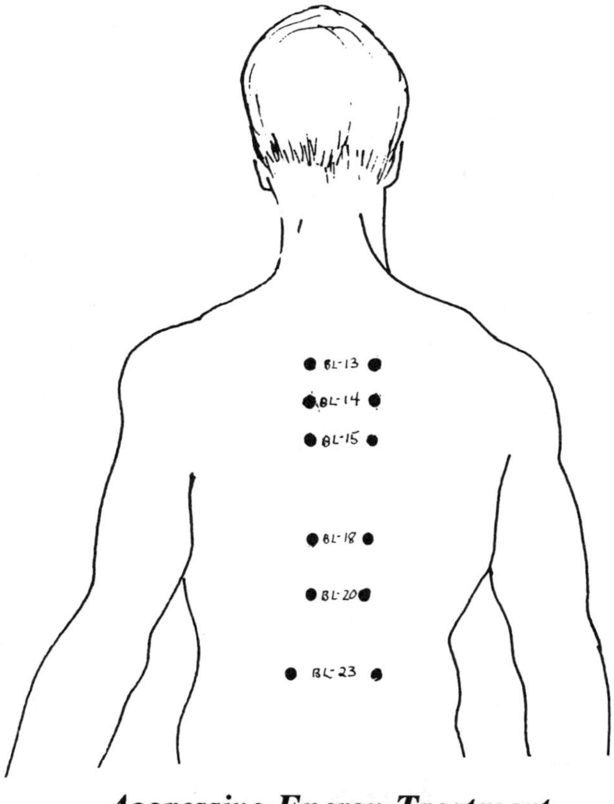

Aggressive Energy Treatment

What about those of you who are unable to find or go to an acupuncturist? If you think you may have Aggressive Energy, my suggestion to you is to have someone sting you on the points illustrated above. It may not be quite as good as an acupuncture treatment, but it's definitely a step in the right direction.

A HUSBAND—WIFE IMBALANCE (H—W)

In general, you will not know if you need this treatment without a trained acupuncturist to assess your pulses, but is worth mentioning because it is a major stumbling block to your health if you have it. The pulses on the left hand are considered to be the Husband and the right hand is the Wife. The Law of Husband and Wife states that the pulses on the left hand (Husband) should be slightly stronger qualitatively and quantitatively than the right hand pulses (the Wife). If this is reversed, it is called a Husband-Wife Imbalance. This is serious and must be corrected immediately. There is a sense of chaos with this condition. The person may feel like they are being torn apart or that they have to give up a part of themselves to survive. The indications for a Husband-Wife Imbalance are:

- Pulse Picture—This is the main indication. The pulses on the left hand (the Husband) are supposed to be stronger qualitatively and quantitatively than the pulses on the right hand (the Wife). In a H—W this would be reversed; the pulses on the right hand will be stronger than the pulses on the left.

- A Bad Marriage/relationship—If it is badly out of balance, they may feel like they have to give up a part of themselves to survive.

- Job—They have a very demanding job and they don't get much out of it. They may say, "This job is killing me!"

- Health—They may be chronically ill and there is chaos to their energy.

- The Bee Venom Therapy does not seem to be working.

- They may feel split and are trying to bring themselves into balance.

Here are the points an acupuncturist would tonify to correct this condition:

KIDNEY-7
BLADDER-67
KIDNEY-3
BLADDER-64
LIVER-3
GALL BLADDER-40
LIVER-4

If the H—W is not broken after doing these points, the practitioner can tonify the following points:

BLADDER-15
BLADDER-18
BLADDER-19
BLADDER-23
BLADDER-27
BLADDER-28

If the H—W is still not broken, then the acupuncturist can sedate the following points: These points should not be stung because bee stings will stimulate or tonify the points rather than sedate them. These points can be massaged with a counter-clockwise motion instead.

LUNG-5
COLON-2
STOMACH-42
SPLEEN-3
HEART PROTECTOR-7
THREE HEATER-4

When the H—W is finally broken, stinging the following two points will keep the imbalance from coming back:

HEART-7
SMALL INTESTINE-4

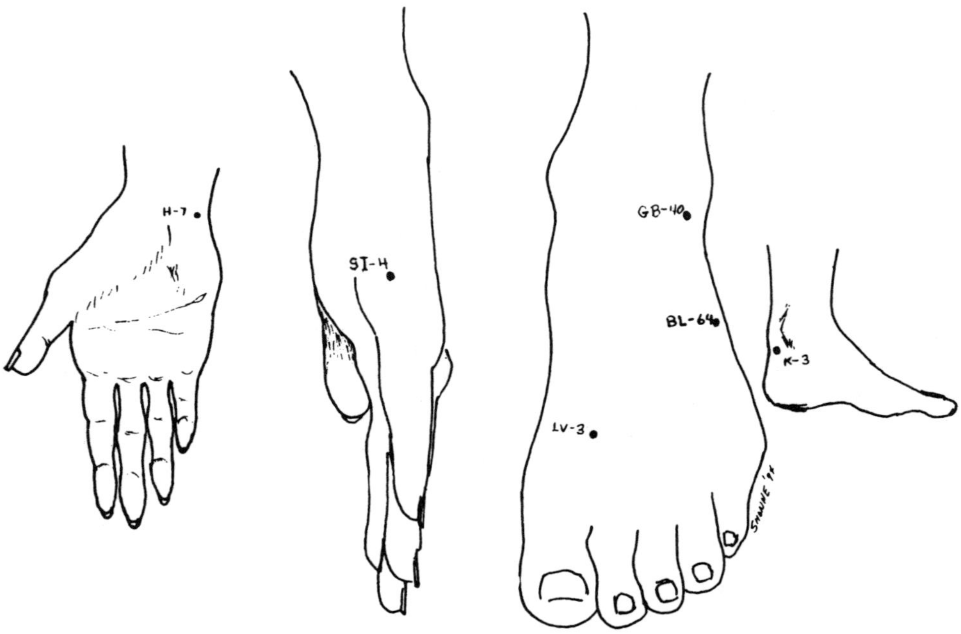

Treatment of Husband—Wife Imbalance

The Chinese pulse picture is very different than the Western pulse picture. As an acupuncturist I am looking at the quantity and quality of the pulse, but I am not counting the number of beats per minute. There are twelve positions (6 on each wrist) to check the pulse for each of the 12 meridians. The goal is to have all pulses in balance and harmony.

Good luck trying to break this major block. I have done it successfully with bees alone and no needles. Just remember that if you do all the points on the feet within the first month or so you may get a great deal of swelling. I would therefore save this treatment until after you are no longer swelling very much on the feet.

WINDOWS OF THE SKY

There are 11 Windows of the Sky. Most of them are on the neck or close to it. A Window is indicated when the person really wants a breakthrough. They have to be ready. They will ask you for it, and even beg for it.

They may say, "I really want to see what happened in my childhood." Or they may say, "I'm at the end of my rope; I have to break through all this soon!" They may also state that they "feel cut off from the neck down."

In general, when we go through a major trauma in childhood, we shut down. In this case, we close down our Windows. Tonifying a Window will help the person to open up more. Windows bring the body, mind and spirit together. You can open up a Window with the bees, because they will tonify the point. If you want to sedate a Window when it's too open, you would probably need to use a needle or use acupressure on the point (the acupuncturist would turn it counter-clockwise). In general I don't recommend trying to sedate a point with bee stings, because (as I stated earlier) the very act of stinging the person will stimulate rather than sedate the point.

The following points are Windows of the Sky:

SMALL INTESTINE-16
SMALL INTESTINE-17
BLADDER -10
HEART PROTECTOR-1 (MEN)(**F** in WOMEN)
HEART PROTECTOR -2 (WOMEN)
THREE HEATER-16
LUNG-3 **F** (acupressure only)
COLON -18
STOMACH-9 **F** (acupressure only)
CONCEPTION VESSEL-22
GOVERNOR VESSEL-16 **F** (acupressure only)

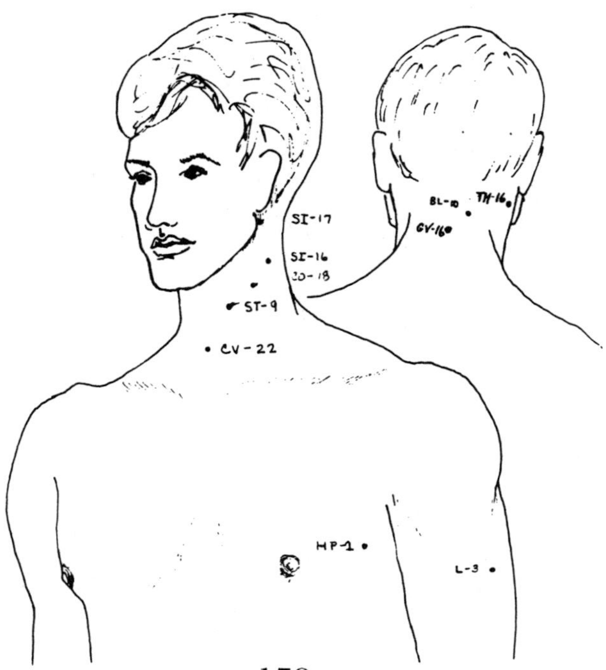

ENTRY/EXIT BLOCK

Each pathway has an entry and an exit point. These points are located at or near the beginning and end of each pathway, and are the points from which the energy flows from one meridian to the next. This energy flows in the same order described in the Chinese Clock. The direction of flow in the Chinese Clock is based on the anatomical relationship between the meridians. The heart pathway, for example, flows from H-1 down the arm to the inside of the little finger, which is the exit point, H-9. The very first point on the small intestine, SI-1, is on the outside of the little finger. The *Ch'i* flows across the nail from H-9 to SI-1, the small intestine entry point. The Chinese Clock thus shows the energy flowing from the heart to the small intestine.

The entry/exit points are like gateways, and can be rusted shut or open. This would be an entry/exit block. It can be easily corrected by treating the entry and exit points on one pathway and perhaps the entry and exit points on the following pathway. By "following pathway," I mean the next pathway according to the Chinese Clock. (See figure at page 58.) There are 12 major pathways through which energy flows in the body. There are 24 hours in a day, therefore each pathway is at its peak for two hours every day. If you are having symptoms at the same time every day, you probably have an entry/exit block. You will need to flush out the pathway.

For example, the time of day that goes with the liver pathway is 1 a.m.—3 a.m. ("sun" time, not daylight savings time). If you are consistently waking up in the middle of the night at this time, it means you have an entry/exit block on the liver. You would need to treat LV-1 and LV-13 and 14 (the liver has two exit points, which is unusual). But if you are waking up at 3:15 a.m. that is in the lung time, so in this case you might want to treat the liver exit points and the entry point on the lungs, L-1. Or here's another very classic pattern: a person who has had a death in the family may wake up at 3 a.m. (the lung time, a time of grief and letting go, feelings of loss). If there is also anger involved, they may wake up at 2 or 2:30 a.m., and not be able to get back to sleep. This is the transition time between anger and grief. This condition indicates an entry/exit block between the liver and the lungs.

What this means is that the energy around the Chinese Clock is not functioning properly. If there is a block on this level, the energy is unable to flow smoothly in its normal path from the exit point of one meridian to the entry point of the next meridian. So a bottleneck, blockage, or excess starts to build up at the exit point. Think of a garden hose with kinks or knots in it. The water cannot flow through it very well and so not much water will come out when you try to water your plants.

This condition can be very frustrating, because no matter what the person does, they can't seem to break the pattern. The condition persists, sometimes for years. Medications to treat the symptoms only cover up the problem like a band-aid. An acupuncturist can correct this block in just a matter of minutes. Now you can see why we ask people what their favorite time of day is and what their worst time of day is. A entry/exit block can be detected on the pulses.

You probably need to use entry/exit points when two or more consecutive pathways are having trouble. In this case consecutive means according to the Chinese Clock. This means that you would have *symptoms* at the *same time* almost every day. You may also need to use entry/exit points when the patient is doing well and then all of a sudden the old symptoms come back.

Here is the list of entry/exit points for each pathway.

	ENTRY	EXIT
	GB-1 take care	GB-41
	LV-1	LV-14 (LV -13)
	H-1	H-9
	SI-1	SI-19
	HP-1 (MEN)	HP-8
	HP-2 (WOMEN)	HP-8
	TH-1	TH-22
F	ST-1	ST-42
	SP-1	SP-21
	L-1	L-7
	CO-4	CO-20 (take care)
F	BL-1	BL-67
	K-1	K-22
	CV-1 (take care)	CV-24 (take care)
	GV-1	GV-28 (take care)

SCARS

Because scars block the flow of energy in the body, they are also considered major blocks. These should be treated by stinging directly on the scar and to either side of the scar. This will promote healing by bringing blood to the area. Also, you can sting the closest acupuncture points above and below the scar. If a scar cuts through a pathway, energy may be blocked.

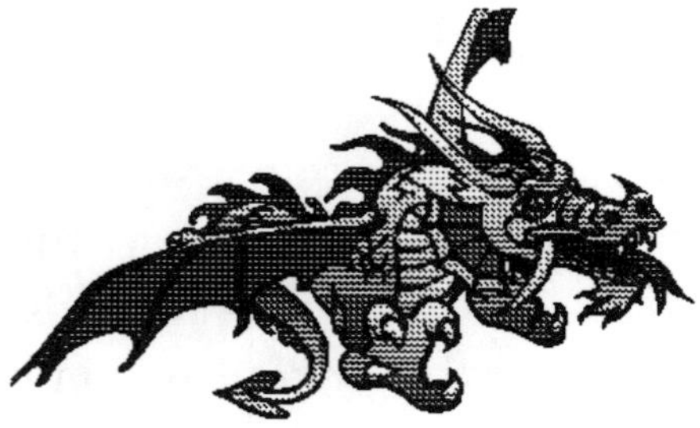

GOOD LUCK, MAY THE DRAGONS BE WITH YOU AS YOU WING YOUR WAY THROUGH THE MAJOR BLOCKS!

PART 3
COMMON SENSE

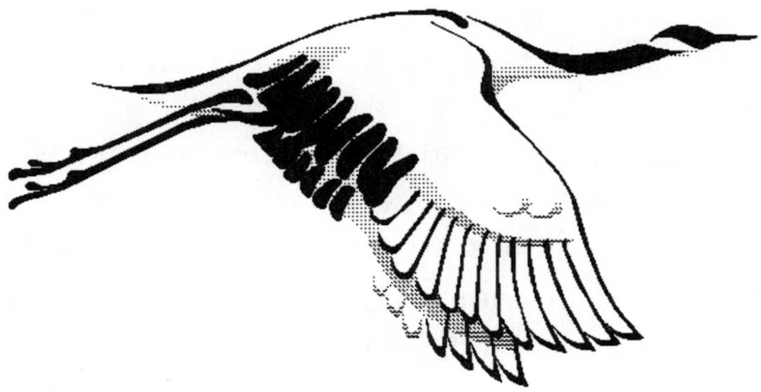

"I PROMISE YOU, IT WON'T HAPPEN AGAIN!"

MARISA'S STORY

I have MS. I began the bee sting therapy in July 1993. The first six times the sting sites became moderately inflamed—a red circle approximately two inches in diameter—with slight to moderate itching. By this time I was getting six stings three times a week.

Early in September after the seventh stinging session, my reaction was quite dramatic. The next day I developed circular welts at each sting site on my right leg of five inches in diameter. The itching was absolutely maddening. My thigh swelled to nearly twice its normal size. I had a fever, and felt "flu-ish" for 3 to 4 days. Even Benadryl would not stop the itching. I tried ice, warm compresses, Preparation H, calamine lotion, all to no avail. It was awful during the day and even worse at night. I called Amber to report the situation. She was very supportive and comforting. She reminded me that this was probably the "healing crisis." I told her that I could not bear the fever, the weakness, and the itching. I was strongly leaning toward discontinuing the therapy even though I had shown improvement in walking, leg movement, and a greatly improved energy level.

Amber encouraged me to speak with another woman who had experienced a similar reaction. She almost gave up because the "healing crisis" was so strong, but she decided to give it another try. She had no reaction the next time. I will never forget her words, "I promise you, it won't happen again." After taking a "rest" for about a week and a half (and noticing an appreciable drop in energy), I worked myself up to trying again. I couldn't believe it. I had no reaction—no swelling, no itching, no fever.

I continue to receive 8 stings every other day. The only reaction I have had since the "healing crisis" is a small red spot at each sting site no larger than a mosquito bite and it fades away in about two hours. I have also had great success stinging a hysterectomy scar. The areas on the scar that I have stung have faded dramatically; the areas that I did not sting have remained the same.

MARISA AND HER HUSBAND TOOK OVER MY PRACTICE (STINGING PEOPLE TWICE A WEEK) WHILE I WAS IN CHINA FOR THREE WEEKS. THEY STILL STING SEVERAL PATIENTS WHO HAVE TROUBLE GETTING TO MY HOME. A.R.

CHAPTER 10

"WHAT DO I DO IF I FEEL THAT I'M NOT GETTING BETTER?"

Healing with bees takes time. It is certainly a common experience for people to become discouraged on occasion, either from the irritation accompanying the stings, or from a feeling that sufficient progress is not being made or sustained. The following list may help you learn how to get "unstuck":

"BEE" patient. You didn't get this way overnight, so you won't get better overnight. You may be tempted to give up too soon because you are in a hurry.

DON'T GIVE UP FIVE MINUTES BEFORE THE MIRACLE!

Comparisons. "How come Pat Wagner is walking and I'm still in my wheelchair?" Please don't compare yourself to anybody else who is doing the bee stings. Everyone's healing process is different. The only person you can compare yourself to is you!

Vitamin C. It is very important to have plenty of Vitamin C while you are doing the bee stings. I cannot stress this enough! Doing bee stings without adequate Vitamin C is like putting high performance gasoline additives in your car but no gas and expecting it to run well. The bee stings stimulate the adrenal glands to produce cortisol, but the adrenal glands need Vitamin C to do this. Our bodies do not make Vitamin C, so we have to get it from an outside source. It is recommended that you take at least 2-3,000 milligrams of Vitamin C every day while doing the bee stings. This is much more than you can get from just drinking orange juice. You may want to consider other vitamins as well: Vitamin B complex, B-12 shots, Vitamin E. If you do take megadoses of Vitamin C, when you discontinue it's a good idea to step down gradually rather than to just stop.

Scars. If you have any scars on your body, it makes it harder for energy to flow through your body. This may interfere with the bee stings. It is recommended that you actually sting yourself on the scar and just to the side of the scar. You may be amazed if you take before and after pictures. I have seen scars completely vanish with bee sting therapy. You can also approach scars from an Oriental point of view. Scars may block the energy in acupuncture pathways. To correct this, sting the closest acupuncture points above and below the scar. This will help restore the flow of energy.

Major Blocks. If you have a major block somewhere on your body, you may not respond as well to the bee stings as others. Think of a garden hose. If you turn the water on and very little water comes out of the hose, it probably means you have a knot somewhere in the hose. You would have to unravel the knot before you could expect to see a difference in the amount of water coming out of the hose. The same is true about energy in the human body. If you have a "knot" or a major block somewhere, it will probably inhibit or prevent the flow of energy. You may want to try acupuncture to correct this. I recommend the following acupuncture treatments for major blocks: the Internal Dragons[G], the External Dragons[G], testing for Aggressive Energy[G], breaking a Husband-Wife Imbalance[G] (when necessary), opening or closing Windows of the Sky[G], or correcting an entry/exit block.[G] These treatments can be done with acupuncture needles by a trained acupuncturist and/or bees. (See Chapter 9 for a description of these Major Blocks.)

Priorities. Although your priority may be to walk well, to get rid of the numbness in your hands, to see or hear better, or to have improved bladder and bowel control, your body may have other priorities. The functioning of the heart muscle and the brain, for example, may take on a larger priority when you view the human machine as a whole.

I urge that you be patient and give the bee stings a good solid try, i.e., six months to a year. Although we are not really sure just how bee venom works, it may be that the energy and sense of well being that often accompanies this therapy may come from the fact that the internal organs are getting what they need. So, if you notice that others are "getting better results" than you are, it may be that you have more repair work that needs to be done.

The visible physical symptoms are often the tip of the iceberg. There are internal physical and spiritual problems as well. I treat the whole person. Be patient as your whole body is healed, not just external physical symptoms.

Indeed, I believe that the increased energy and sense of well-being that often occurs is due to the healing of your internal organs. The largest part of healing is internal (invisible). We are not always aware of what's going on inside.

Just as a candlestick may be so badly tarnished that its true beauty is not visible, you may be so involved with your symptoms that you don't see the possibility of your healing. Polish does not make the candlestick beautiful. The polish only allows the candlestick's beauty to shine. Similarly, bee stings don't cure anything. They stimulate your body to heal itself. Your health is just below the surface. You may have to dig for it, but it's been there all along.

The Number of Stings. Pat Wagner suggests that if you feel you are at a plateau and you want to get a "boost" or a "lift," temporarily increase the number of stings that you get. For example, if you are used to doing 20 stings each time, go up to 30 stings for two sessions and then go back to 20 stings and see what happens. Conversely, if you are doing 40 stings without much change over time, try decreasing the number for a while. You can always go back up.

Nutrition. Proper nutrition is an important part of your healing process. Read some books on nutrition. (See Appendix II.) I recommend minimizing the amount of sugar, dairy, fat, and white flour products in your diet. Alcohol and cigarettes also block the benefits of bee sting therapy. (See Chapter 12 on Nutrition and Food Allergies.)

Allergies. Food allergies may be affecting your healing. If you think you are allergic to some foods, try eliminating them from your diet. You can also have your blood tested for food allergies. I have often found that the bee stings are more effective after allergic foods are eliminated from the diet. (For additional information, see Chapter 12.)

Medications. It is harder for the bee stings to work when you're taking a lot of medicine. If your goal is to slowly come off the medication, that's great. Medication could reduce the healing impact of the stings. Be sure to consult with your physician before you adjust or eliminate any prescribed medications!

Rest. Make sure your body is getting enough rest. Listen to your body! If you are doing too much, your body will tell you. Respect your body, hear its wisdom, and accommodate its needs.

Exercise. Exercise is very important. Find the form that is right for you: bicycling, stretching, yoga, swimming. Yes, you can do exercises even if you are in a wheelchair. Consider physical therapy if you think it might be beneficial.

Reconnect Spiritually. Consider trying prayer and/or meditation. Find a Higher Power, try going to a support group, or try saying the serenity prayer to yourself:

GOD, GRANT ME THE SERENITY
TO ACCEPT THE THINGS I CANNOT CHANGE
THE COURAGE TO CHANGE THE THINGS I CAN
AND THE WISDOM TO KNOW THE DIFFERENCE

Reach out to others. Call a friend, or find something meaningful to do. Reach out to someone else who is having a hard time. You may want to try stinging somebody else.

Giving is an important part of your healing. Realize that no matter what you are dealing with, you have something precious to share. By giving, you create room for more good in your life. Share the love and energy that you have received. Healing is a circle, a giving circle. Everything you give comes back to you multiplied.

Goals. Finish a project that was left half started. Try to remember what your goals were before you got this disease. Can you still complete those goals in some form? Or is it time to reassess and set new ones?

"Get a Life." What else is going on in your life? Is something left unresolved? What do you need to accept that you may be resisting? What can you do to change your attitude or your part in the situation?

If you could wave a magic wand, what would you wish for? Think about what is getting in your way. Ask yourself "What am I doing on this planet?" Do you remember what you came here to do? It's never too late to follow your dream. Only you can write the next "chapter" of your life. GO FOR IT!

"Accentuate the Positive." Focus on what you can do, rather than what you can't do. Work on letting go of negative thoughts and situations. You cannot control people, places and things. The only thing you can change is yourself and how you respond to your experiences.

Make a Gratitude List. Make a list of all the important people in your life. Make a list of all the things that you are grateful for. Count your blessings.

Have Fun! Think of three things that you enjoy doing and do them! Do some things that make you laugh. Remember, it's never too late for a happy childhood.

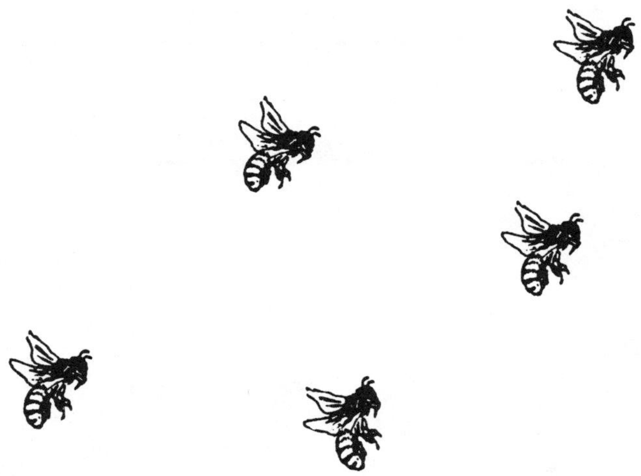

AERODYNAMICALLY, IT IS IMPOSSIBLE FOR A HONEYBEE TO FLY. MODERN SCIENCE BELIEVES THAT HER BODY IS TOO HEAVY TO BE CARRIED BY HER FRAGILE WINGS . . . AND YET SHE FLIES!

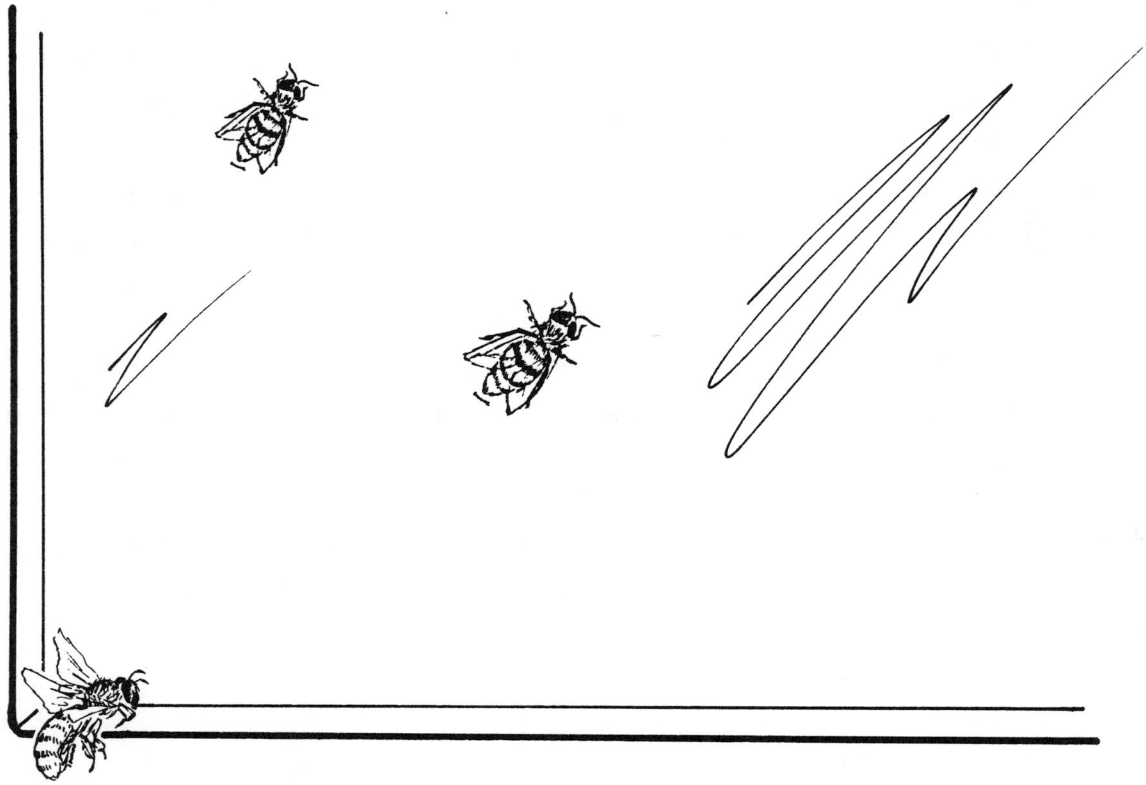

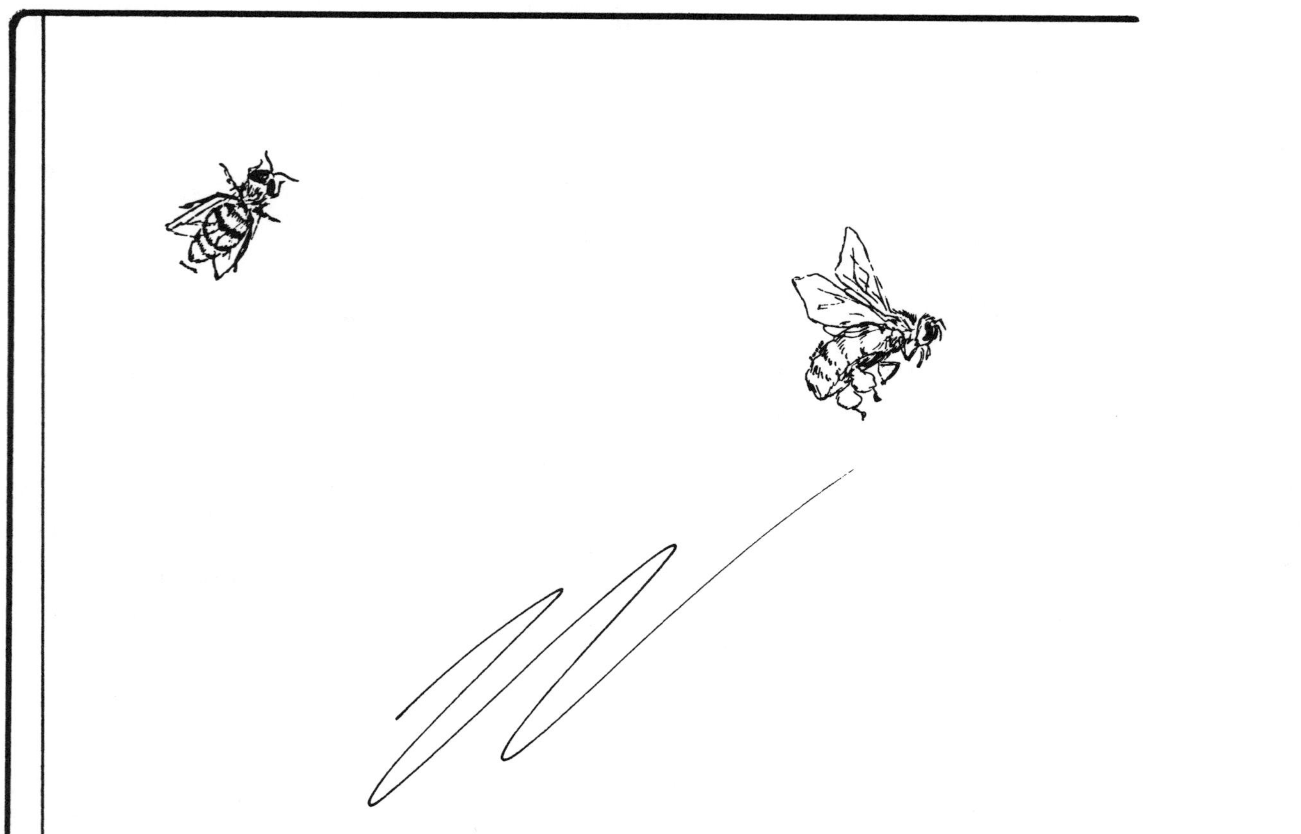

CHAPTER 11

IF YOU ARE STINGING SOMEONE ELSE

CONGRATULATIONS! You have conquered your fear of bees, or you are stretching in that direction. BRAVO!

Here are some important things to remember:

COPING WITH THE STINGS:

The person you are helping may swell, itch, and get red during the first month or so. Not only is this normal, but this is a good sign, because it means that the person's immune system is waking up.

Remember you can use ice or an ice pack before and after the stings to reduce the pain. I also recommend Preparation-H (or a generic brand) to soothe the stings. It seems to work better for me than any anti-histamine. Some people recommend vinegar.

The person you are stinging may get discouraged and want to give up. They need your help and encouragement, especially during "the healing crisis" and if the itching is very bad.

By the way, you can treat accidental stings topically with ammonia if you can get to it during the first minute. Don't use this for intentional stings, as it will curtail the effectiveness of the sting.

APPROACHING TREATMENT:

Involve the person (as much as you can) in the treatment process. Be a good listener and ask them what they need. Remember, the patient has the answers.

Remember, there is a difference between the patient and the story. The symptoms are just information. Be like "an empty bowl" as you are listening to them. You are a "source point[G]" (an acupuncture point that brings the patient the most perfect energy) in the treatment room. Your "intention" is very important. What is it that you are intending to do? Be focused. If you are treating an entry-exit[G] block, then picture it in your mind. You are opening the exit point of one pathway and the entry point of the next pathway. Imagine that you are doing a "roto-rooter" treatment, unclogging the pipes like a plumber. This treatment is very good for those people who are having symptoms at the same time every day. (See glossary[G] for more details.) You can also treat by the spirit of the point, which means that you are picking the point because the name of the point calls out to you. One example of this would be choosing Gate of Hope, Liver 14. This point is good if the person is feeling hopeless and cannot see a future for himself. If you are doing this point for someone, visualize hope or a light at the end of the tunnel. Such visualization gives intention to your act. Don't just sting mechanically, but be conscious of what you are giving.

Remember a very important piece of information: it may serve the patient to keep his or her symptoms. Change is scary. We all want to get well, but sometimes things get in the way. "Bee" patient with those you are helping.

A change in the person is more important than a change in the symptom!!!! This is very, very important.

HEALING IS CONTAGIOUS!

Remember most of all, that healing takes time. Healing is a process and not just a destination. Healing for the patient is something that she creates herself with God's help or Nature's help.

PUTTING THE FIVE ELEMENTS INTO ACTION

Study the five elements carefully yourself. Try to understand yourself and the other person as best you can. The patient is telling you in a thousand ways what they need. They are also disguising in a thousand ways what they need. Do they need some fire today? Is their wood out of balance? Is it spring and therefore would it help to do a horary[G] treatment on the wood element. This is a special treatment which relates to the right time of day or the right season. (See the glossary[G] for a more detailed description.) If you think it would help, stay up to 12:30 a.m. and do a gall bladder horary point and then a liver point after 1:00 a.m. Remember to go by the sun time, not daylight savings time! By the way, even if your gall bladder was removed, you still have a gall bladder pathway.

If you want, you can do acupuncture without needles. You can do acupuncture with your words. Here are some examples:

According to Oriental Philosophy, there are five basic elements in nature: WOOD, FIRE, EARTH, METAL AND WATER. (See Chapter 5 for more details.)

When the wood element is out of balance for a person, he or she may feel: angry, impatient, frustrated, or hopeless. This person needs a plan, a sense of direction, and hope. If, instead, you give them sympathy, "Oh honey, this must be so hard for you!," then you are giving them the emotion that goes with the earth element and they will probably push you away. If you give them love, "Oh, honey, I just love you so much!," then you are giving them the fire element, and they will probably reject it. If you give them respect, "Oh, honey, I respect you so much for trying to help yourself!," you are giving them the metal element and they cannot accept this either. And if you give them reassurance, "Oh, honey, don't worry, everything is going to be OK!," then you are giving them the water element and they may get angry. But if you understand that they need the wood element, and therefore they need a plan, a sense of direction and hope, you have a much better chance of reaching them and making a difference. If you can help them find what they so desperately need, I guarantee you that they will be eternally grateful.

So, if you know which element is the most out of balance (See Chapter 6), you can use your words to give your patient what they really need. That is why it is so important to be a good listener. Don't just look at the symptoms. Remember, they are only part of the whole picture. Look at the whole person. Imagine what they would be like if they were healthy.

Try to be flexible and give the patient what he or she really needs. You, yourself, may be a caretaker type of personality (EARTH) and your natural tendency may be to give a lot of sympathy. They may reject it. Try not to take this personally. Remember, don't give them what you would need if you were sick. Give them what they need!

> HEALING GOES BEYOND THE SYMPTOMS, BEYOND THE PERSON, TO THE FAMILY AND COMMUNITY . . .

If you get angry or impatient, remember you are expressing the wood element. A patient needing sympathy will feel very misunderstood. A patient needing love will feel very unloved. A patient needing respect and appreciation may feel very cut off and isolated. And a patient needing reassurance may feel very afraid of your anger.

This may be a stretch for you, but you can do it! Please don't give up five minutes before the miracle.

HANDLING OBSTACLES:

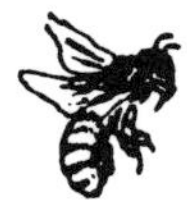

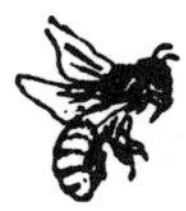

If you do not see much change in the person or if you think you have hit a plateau, read Chapter 10 entitled: "What do I do if I feel like I'm not getting better?" Is the person taking enough Vitamin C, royal jelly, pollen, bee propolis, etc.? Are there any scars that might be blocking the treatments? Are there any major blocks? Can you and/or the patient go to a support group of some kind? What about food allergies or nutrition? What about medication? Could it be blocking your progress together? Try saying the Serenity Prayer. Remember, you are asking for the serenity to accept the things you cannot change (that means people, places and things); the courage to change the things you can (that means yourself, you are the only person you can really change); and the wisdom to know the difference. *Remember also that patients often forget how bad they were before starting the bee stings and then think that they haven't made any progress.*

If you are feeling confused, feel free to write or call someone who is more experienced. Most people who have been doing apitherapy for a while have a wealth of information. Be sure to thank them for their time and be sensitive to the fact that they are probably very busy and may not have a lot of free time to talk. You may want to consider giving a donation for their time and energy.

Remember, it is OK not to have all the answers. Don't be afraid to reach out for help. Those of us who sting others have been where you are now and have probably felt everything you are feeling now.

If you are an apitherapist who finds him or herself stinging many people, it is good to encourage them to take an active part in their treatment. Independence in bee stinging is an important goal. Your "patients" should be encouraged to be active partners and get involved in the process. In my own experience, I've noted a real difference among patients. Some:

- Come to me and I do everything.
- Come to me and I sting them but they bring tweezers, tissues, toilet paper rolls . . . etc.
- Pick up bees from me in a jar . . . and sting themselves 1-3 times per week.
- Get themselves a veil and start collecting bees from my hive and sting themselves at home.
- Get their own bee hives and sting themselves at home.
- Have a beehive at home, sting themselves . . . and then start doing what I'm doing . . . stinging others.

UNDERSTANDING THE SPIRIT OF ILLNESS:

Now, consider the following meditation: God's medicine is life. (And the side effects can be "positive" or "negative.") Then consider this idea:

God sends the illness . . . and then God cures the illness. (We as practitioners are merely instruments through which the healing takes place. We are like farmers, helping nature by getting the rocks out of the soil, planting seeds, watering those seeds . . . and making sure the conditions are right. The patient's illness is a wake up call.)

Now ponder the following: You can find God in the illness! If this is true, it would inspire us to make a medicine out of the illness. Respect the illness, give it meaning. This is what healing is all about.

Look to see what is showing up as missing. Look for an opening. When you have isolation with illness, life becomes meaningless. Empower the person you are working with. And if there is fear with the illness, bring faith . . . because when fear knocks and faith answers, there is no soil in which the fear and its ill-effects can take root.

Treat your patients with more than needles or bees, treat them with your heart. If you know how to ask the right questions, and you can listen well, you will understand your patients, not only with your mind, but with your heart.

I'd like to leave you with one last thought: Remember that all true healing happens spirit to spirit. While you need to keep your own center and not assume responsibility for those who are ill, the real miracle happens when you become one with your patients.

IF I DON'T KNOW WHO YOU ARE

I SERVE YOU

BUT IF I KNOW WHO YOU ARE

I AM YOU

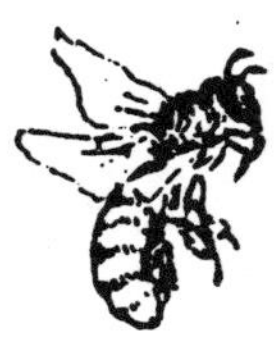

CHAPTER 12

NUTRITION AND FOOD ALLERGIES

Hippocrates, the Father of Western Medicine, said in 400 B.C.: "Thy food shall be thy remedy." The proper foods can cleanse, restore and nourish the body. Libraries and bookstores have hundreds of books on nutrition. I encourage you to study those books which appeal to you. You may find contradictory theories. Don't be discouraged; there is no one diet that works for everyone. There are no panaceas.

There is an inherent irony in the idea that "Food is your Best Medicine" (Bieler). If you are allergic to certain foods, they can also become your "enemy." If you know which foods are enemies and which are friends, then the solution is simple. You stay away from your enemies and remain close to your friends. For example, if you know that you are allergic to poison ivy, you don't roll around in it. It is the same with food. If you know you are allergic to dairy products, avoid them. Common allergies include: milk and all dairy products, sugar, wheat, corn, yeast, alcohol, chocolate and caffeine.

Food allergies are more common than many realize. I believe that when the immune system is suppressed or not functioning properly, the body may have abnormal reactions to foods that would not bother a healthy person. If you pay attention to your body, you may notice, for example, that you always get a headache or feel tired after eating a certain food. This is important information and should not be ignored. Sometimes the very foods that you love and crave are the ones to which you are allergic. It is also possible to become addicted to certain foods and get symptoms when you don't eat them. This is called a "masked allergy." It is similar to withdrawal symptoms from drugs. One woman I know says that chocolate is the only thing that cures her headaches. But it may be that the headache is a "withdrawal symptom" and eating the chocolate stops the symptom temporarily.

There is a blood test for allergies. The ELIZA/ACT test (Enzyme-Linked Immunosorbent Assay/Advanced Cell Test) helps identify both immediate-type and delayed-type food allergies. This test may be able to detect 70-80% of the foods to which you are allergic. You may want to ask your doctor about this test.

To learn more, read Dr. Robert Soll's book, "MS: Something Can Be Done and You Can Do It!" (See the Reading List in Appendix II.)

You can also test yourself for food allergies. This do-it-yourself approach is discussed in Judy Graham's book, "Multiple Sclerosis, a Self-Help Guide to its Management." She recommends starting with a cleansing fast. Then, you introduce the foods one by one to see if they cause a reaction.

Intestinal Candida can be a major cause of food allergies. Candida Albicans yeast grows in and on most people. It is usually controlled by the immune system. When the body's immune system is suppressed, this yeast may continue to grow uncontrolled. The by-products of the yeast colonies are absorbed into the bloodstream. These toxins can be carried by the blood and spread throughout the body. Hence, it is thought that people with Candida have symptoms in many areas of the body. Examples of common Candida symptoms include: vaginal yeast infections, chronic fatigue, severe menstrual cramps, bloating, diarrhea, headaches, asthma, bladder infections, skin problems and depression. (See the Reading List for books on Candida. Pay special attention to "The Yeast Connection" by Dr. Crook, "The Yeast Syndrome" by Dr. John Trowbridge, and "The Body Ecology Diet" by Donna Gates. These books contain diet suggestions and helpful recipes.)

Certain drugs appear to increase a person's sensitivity to Candida. These include: antibiotics (which change the delicate bacteria balance in the body), birth control pills (which suppress the immune system), sulfanomide drugs, steroids, and immunosuppressive drugs (which are often given to people who already have something wrong with their immune system). Some drugs properly used can be powerful allies, but many drugs do more harm than the original disease.

Many physicians are in a state of "drug hypnosis." They apparently believe nature must be assisted by their laboratory concoctions. This misuse of drugs and lack of respect for Mother Nature is not new. About 100 years ago Dr. Oliver Wendell Holmes wrote:

> "I firmly believe if the whole 'materia medica' as now used could be sunk to the bottom of the sea, it would be all the better for mankind —and all the worse for the fishes."

The constant over-use of prescription drugs has created what is now called iatrogenic disease—illnesses induced in a patient by a doctor's actions. I believe drugs often suppress the body's natural healing powers and drive the illness deeper.

The following example illustrates the danger of treating symptoms. A man had eczema. Medicines eventually made the eczema disappear, but he then developed lung problems, including wheezing. His doctor prescribed a new medicine which stopped the wheezing. Within a few months the patient developed pleurisy. Antibiotics were then prescribed for the pleurisy. The pleurisy went away. He eventually developed bronchitis and asthma. He lived with this chronic condition for many years.

So, something that started out as a skin problem became asthma over the years. In Chinese medicine the skin is considered the third lung. On the case mentioned above, as the disease is treated symptomatically on the outside of the body (the skin), it is driven deeper inside the body (the lungs).

This is a very important concept. As you begin to heal yourself, you may experience prior symptoms in reverse order. A patient being treated for asthma may develop bronchitis, pleurisy, wheezing, eczema or some other skin ailment before becoming well. This is called the Law of Cure. It is important to realize that the patient is really being healed although the symptoms may appear to be getting worse.

Hippocrates was convinced that poisonous and potent drugs were not the means to restore health. The world's greatest physicians used but a few simple drugs. Hippocrates knew the importance of nature in the healing process. He prescribed good wholesome food, rest, sleep, fresh air, recreation, physiotherapy and change of climate so that the body's wisdom and nature could do the real healing.

You may think of your body as a "Do-It-Yourself Repair Kit." Good nutritious foods are the "raw materials" or "parts" your body uses to heal itself.

The following guidelines will help you to become your own nutritionist and increase your good judgment as you select the foods that are right for you:

✓ It's best to get your nutrition with a "fork and a spoon." Ideally your food should be your medicine. Today's food is not as good as the food our grandparents ate. It is too often deficient in nutrients and filled with pesticides, hormones, antibiotics and other additives. You may consider using vitamin and mineral supplements, and whole food herbal concentrates. The best herbal food concentrates I've seen are put out by Sunrider International. (See Appendix II for directions to order Sunrider Herbal Foods.)

✓ Eat foods that are as close as possible to their raw or whole food state. Locally grown foods in season are best. Eat lots of fresh fruits, vegetables, and whole grains. Avoid highly processed foods. If you think you may have candida, stay away from fruits, sweets, yeast, etc. (See the Reading List for books on diet information for candida.)

✓ Variety is the spice of life. Don't eat the same foods every day.

✓ Eat small, frequent meals. You will feel better and have more energy.

✓ Protein is important. You can estimate your protein requirement by dividing your weight by 2.2. For example, a 130 pound person requires 59 grams of protein daily. Too much protein can be as harmful as too little.

✓ Avoid nutritional pitfalls: junk food, sugar, white flour products, chemical food additives, processed oils and fats, saturated fats, caffeine, alcohol, and salt. Not all foods are "created" equal, some are better for you than others. For example, not all fats are bad. Saturated fats are not healthy, but essential fatty acids are very important. (See the Reading List for Professor Swank's book on low-fat diets.)

✓ Drink good water. Consider using bottled water or a good filter. Your body is mostly water. Be sure to drink enough water (8-10 glasses a day).

✓ Air pollution is a serious problem. Consider using an air filter.

Here are some additional thoughts you may want to keep in mind:

✓ The goal of medicine should be to prevent disease, prolong life and improve the quality of one's life. The ideal of medicine is to eliminate the need of a physician. Did you know that in ancient China doctors were only paid when the patient was well, not sick?

✓ A good nutritional program provides you with better disease resistance.

✓ Make nutrition your ally and not your enemy.

✓ Food is like gasoline, high and low octane. The more nutrition in the food, the better it is for you.

✓ Sometimes the key is not what you eat, but what you don't eat. Other times it's not what you eat, but what's eating you.

✓ Nature doesn't follow the Madison Avenue hype of Feel Better Faster. Nature heals slowly. Nature never rushes healing. If an animal is sick, it doesn't eat or drink until it has passed through the worst of the illness and has become stabilized.

✓ Given the opportunity and proper conditions, nature is the greatest healer.

✓ The more involved you are in your healing process, the better the results. Don't give your power to your doctor. Take your health back into your own hands. Be empowered.

Healing takes time. One of your biggest lessons is patience. You are exactly where you are supposed to be right now. Healing doesn't happen overnight. You can't just go to a fast food restaurant (or a doctor's office) and order health. This is your life, not an instant hamburger. Drugs promise immediate relief of symptoms without treating the deeper illness. You are about to embark on the adventure of creating your own health plan. This is a gradual process. You will learn to listen to your body as you try different foods and techniques. Books can only give you ideas. Remember, you are innately your own healer.

CHAPTER 13

OTHER SUGGESTIONS

You may want to explore a number of avenues to round out your healing experience. This chapter is meant to be a smorgasbord featuring a variety of healing methods, the goal being to give you a taste of each technique without going into great depth. The Reading List in the Appendix will provide you with names of books that explain these concepts further. The best book I have seen that compares to an encyclopedia of alternative healing is "Alternative Medicine, The Definitive Guide," compiled by the Burton Goldberg Group. It defines all types of healing methods, gives a list of recommended books on each therapy and supplies you with helpful addresses for programs in your area. Another helpful book by the same publisher is the "Alternative Medicine Yellow Pages."

The following list sets forth a number of HEALING APPROACHES which are available from a trained professional. Following that list are a number of ideas for you to consider doing ON YOUR OWN.

HEALING APPROACHES:

ACUPUNCTURE

This is a Traditional Chinese technique, over 3-5,000 years old, that employs the use of very fine needles to puncture the skin. The goal is to release internal blocks and bring balance and harmony to the body, mind and spirit. The Chinese believed that energy (*Ch'i*) flows through the body along twelve basic pathways or meridians. These pathways are associated with certain organs in the body and the functions of those organ systems. There are acupuncture points on these pathways that can be stimulated to enhance the flow of *Ch'i*. This corrects the flow of energy in the body, reduces pain, and restores health to the patient. A traditional acupuncturist may prescribe herbal formulas or use herbs directly/indirectly on the body, a technique called moxibustion.

BODYWORK

Bodywork is a variety of therapies which increase deep relaxation, alleviate or reduce pain, ease injured muscles, increase lymphatic circulation, and increase blood flow. Here are some examples of different kinds of bodywork: Acupressure, Shiatsu, Therapeutic Massage, Therapeutic Touch, Rolfing, Feldenkrais Method, Reflexology, Polarity Therapy, Trager Therapy, and Bonnie Prudden Myotherapy.

CHELATION THERAPY

This is a treatment which can be safe and effective for many people. It is a method for drawing metabolic waste and toxins out of the bloodstream. This can be done through either intravenous or oral methods. Either method should be administered or monitored by a physician. Some conditions that may benefit from chelation therapy include: cardiac arrhythmia, atherosclerosis, and problems with memory, concentration, and vision.

CHIROPRACTIC

This therapeutic system regards many disease processes as the result of subluxations (misalignments) of the spine. A Chiropractor manipulates or adjusts subluxations of the spinal column and other structures to promote health and relieve pain. Chiropractic has a profound effect on the nervous system (because the nerves come out of the spine) and on the body's own natural mechanisms of defense. Chiropractic extends as far back as Egyptian times and it is practiced in many civilizations. Daniel David Palmer founded in 1895 what we have come to know as modern-day Chiropractic.

HOLISTIC DENTISTRY—AMALGAM REMOVAL

Mercury toxicity may result from the amalgam fillings in your teeth leaking toxins into your body. The presence of mercury, tin, copper, silver, and zinc may make it difficult for you to get well. While the extent of this problem remains somewhat unclear, research coming out of Europe suggests that modern-day dentistry contributes to chronic diseases (indirectly or directly). It is often highly recommended to have one's mercury based fillings removed from the mouth and replaced with non-toxic, filling material. Using a dentist experienced in this technique is critical; this process can temporarily make things worse, as some of the mercury in the fillings is released during its removal.

It is also interesting to note that Reinhold Voll, M.D. discovered in the 1950's that every tooth in the mouth corresponds to a specific acupuncture pathway, and therefore a specific organ system in the body.

HOMEOPATHY

This is a unique system of medicine that is based on the belief that "like cures like." Homeopathy was started by Hahnemann, a famous German physician in the late 1700's. He discovered through trial and error that substances that produce symptoms when given in large doses often instigate a curative reaction for those same symptoms when given in small doses. Hahnemann believed that the more the substance is diluted the more powerful the remedy. In other words, a homeopathic physician prescribes remedies that use extremely small quantities of plants, minerals, or animals, that if used in larger doses would produce similar symptoms of the disease that is being treated. The remedies come in the following four forms: granules, powder, tablets, and tincture. You place the remedies under your tongue; do not touch the remedies with your hands or take them before or after a meal.

NATUROPATHIC MEDICINE (NATUROPATHY)

Naturopathy is a compilation of healing practices that work together to heal the Body, Mind and Spirit. Widely known for its "drugless therapies," it draws on folk remedies that have been practiced all over the world for thousands of years, as well as modern scientific techniques. Naturopathy places an emphasis on treating the underlying cause of disease using nutrition, herbs, and other remedies. Its foundation is based on six basic philosophies that have been tested over time: 1) First, do no harm; 2) Treat the cause rather than the symptom; 3) Treat the whole person; 4) The body will heal itself when given a chance; 5) The physician should be a teacher; and 6) The best cure is prevention.

OSTEOPATHY

Osteopathy is a medical therapy which combines Western medical approaches with a focus on correcting problems of the musculo-skeletal system of the body through soft-tissue manipulations. The first school of Osteopathy was founded in Kirksville, Missouri in 1892, by a registered physician named Dr. Andrew Taylor Still. Osteopathy is helpful in treating chronic diseases and pain, but it also looks for the deeper problems underlying the illness. Osteopathy uses some of the following techniques as part of its therapy: cranial manipulation, muscle energy work, soft tissue work, techniques to reduce muscular spasms, and gentle mobilization.

ON YOUR OWN:

ATTITUDE

Your mental attitude has a direct impact on your health. A positive attitude can turn an obstacle into a stepping stone. Negative thoughts can erode your health and slow down your healing process. Depression is usually anger turned inward and is only solved through action. You may want to consider finding a professional counselor to work through some of your emotional issues. If you bottle up your emotions your body will pay the price. There are many ways to work on improving your self-esteem and your attitude, such as prayer, support groups, self-help books, affirmations and visualization techniques. Another way to brighten your day is to reach out to others who are having a hard time. Remember, even if you are in a wheelchair, you can still reach out to others who need your support. Sometimes a smile and a kind word will make a big difference. Part of getting well is giving to others.

BACH FLOWER REMEDIES

This is the use of extracted plant/flower oils to alter human emotions such as anger, lack of joy, worry, grief and fear. The patient's emotional state determines the remedy selected. There is a questionnaire that allows you to select the remedy which relates to you. For example, those people who feel a lot of guilt and tend to blame themselves for everything would be encouraged to try "Pine."

The most famous remedy from this collection is called Rescue Remedy and is for emergency situations. These remedies were based on the theories of Dr. Edward Bach, a British Physician in the early 1930's. He believed that the body's lack of resistance to disease was connected to negative emotional states. The essences of the flowers assist in alleviating these negative states. There are flower essences available from other sources as well as those developed by Dr. Bach.

BREATHING TECHNIQUES

Breathing is a very important part of one's health. Breathing is the only physical function which is subject to both voluntary and autonomic control. Taking control of your breath can have profound effects. Deep breathing exercises will help you relax and improve your emotional outlook. It is hard to breath deeply and be tense at the same time. There are a variety of breathing techniques that are practiced in Yoga. Rebirthing is another way of using the breath to experience awareness and focus on positive affirmations.

EXERCISE

Exercise is very important for many reasons. It improves the circulation and immune function, keeps the muscles strong, increases your energy, and may in some cases lift depression. Exercises can even be done by people in wheelchairs. You can do exercises at home or in the office of a physical therapist. It is ideal for you to do some sort of exercise every other day. A good exercise program can reduce stress and have beneficial effects on the physical body. It is also important to note that exercising too much can cause stress and wear out the body. An exercise program should be designed to be appropriate to the individuals needs and limitations.

MEDITATION

Meditation is a way to clear yourself of daily trivia and calm your mind. It helps you keep your attention on the present moment. It is often done in a sitting position where you concentrate on one thing only; this could be a single thought, a chant, a "mantra," or even just your breath. When done every day meditation helps you stay calm and centered. It reduces stress and allows you to relax. It helps you develop a deeper sense of control over your life.

There are other kinds of meditations where you bring awareness to your life. Walking Meditation involves intentionally experiencing the sensations of walking. You pay attention to the way your body moves as you are walking. In a more informal way you can meditate while you are washing the dishes or cleaning the house. You can pay attention to your breathing and calm your mind. Any activity can become a form of meditation. An old Buddhist saying is, "When carrying water, I am carrying water." In other words, you are *only* carrying water, not arguing in your head with the kids or figuring out how to pay the bills. By being fully in the present, you get out of your body's way and let it relax and heal.

RELAXATION

There are many relaxation techniques such as hypnosis, guided imagery, and visualizations. These may prove to be very helpful to you, but what's most important is you finding ways to relax or taking the time to do things you enjoy, such as taking a bubble bath, reading a good book, calling a friend, being out in nature, listening to music you love, doing something creative, enjoying your own company, living in the moment (not holding onto the past or worrying about the future), and taking care of yourself.

YOGA

Yoga is a system of exercise and meditation that is practiced in order to promote control of the body and mind, as well as training one's consciousness for a state of perfect spiritual insight and peace. Yoga is a Sanskrit word that means "uniting the self with the universe." It is best if you can go to a Yoga class rather than just trying to learn it from a book. Yoga is more of a total philosophy rather than just a group of exercises. It involves correct breathing and a good positive attitude. Yoga stills the mind and helps the body's own self-healing powers. There are many different kinds of Yoga and many different health conditions that can benefit from its practice.

❧ CONCLUSION ❧

"PEOPLE HELPING PEOPLE"

I dreamt one night that the Great Wall of China led right to my door. ❧ And as I felt the sensation of my feet walking across the wall, I realized that the Wall had become a bridge from West to East and East to West: a bridge across cultures, instead of a Great Wall to keep out the enemy.

It has become clear to me that apitherapy can be a bridge between people. ❧ It's all about a movement of people helping people. ❧ And so many people know about it now, that there's no turning back. ❧ Interest in BVT will go forward. ❧ When there is a critical mass of people excited about it, BVT will be raised from its "folk remedy status."

Some doctors may be threatened by this grassroots movement, but I believe it is time to tear down the "Great Wall" that stands between doctors and patients. ❧ There are no enemies. ❧ A "Great Wall" need not exist. ❧ It's time to transform the wall into a bridge between doctors and patients, a bridge that encourages real dialogue and healing.

When the doctor and patient sit together in a treatment room, the real knowledge often comes, not from the degree on the wall, but from the experience of having the disease. I honestly believe that if the tables were turned and the doctor had the disease (for example, MS), he or she might be trying bee stings too!

There are times when we are looking for answers in all the wrong places. ❧ Sometimes doctors may have the very answers we need, but other times the answers will be "in our own backyard." ❧ This is one of those times. ❧ It is time to take our health back into our own hands.

I believe it is no coincidence that apitherapy has sprung up naturally in so many cultures. ❧ There is a universal truth here, an example of a healing method drawn from what Carl Jung called the "collective unconscious." ❧ Let us not ignore this important message.

I sincerely believe that BVT, apitherapy, "bee-acupuncture," "honey-bee healing" or "living acupuncture," is as natural as nature itself. ❧ It is surely a gift from God. ❧ It is God's medicine. ❧

A honeybee hive is a virtual medicine chest of health: bee venom, raw honey, pollen, propolis, royal jelly and beeswax. ❧ Any home with a beehive has a "gold mine" in its backyard.

The "gold rush" has already begun. ❧ People are swarming to beekeepers in search of the gold in their hives. ❧ Beekeepers, be open minded. ❧ If you are not comfortable sharing your bees with strangers in wheelchairs, encourage them to get a hive of their own. ❧ Let's start a whole new generation of beekeepers!

With constantly rising health costs, it's time to go back to nature. ❧ Maybe it's time to look in our own backyard. ❧ And maybe it's time to remember the era of the Good Samaritan and the Golden Rule. ❧ People helping people, not just when an earthquake hits, but any time someone needs our help.

Yes, people helping people. ❧ Remember Charlie Mraz and Pat Wagner? ❧ You wouldn't be reading this book if it weren't for them. ❧ I wouldn't have written this book if it weren't for them. ❧ One person can truly make a difference! You can make a difference!

We're all in this together, folks. ❧ People helping people, isn't that what life is all about?

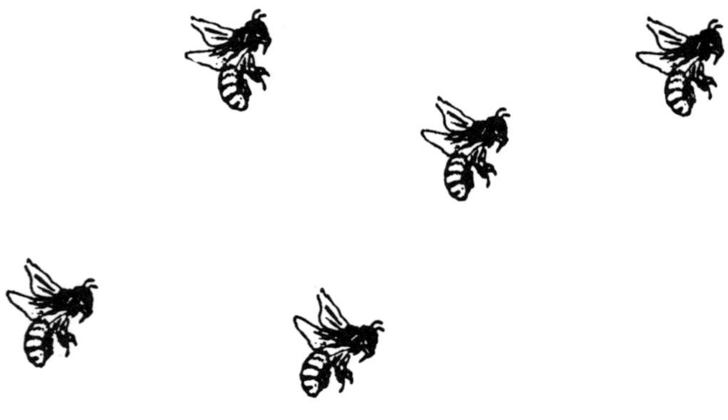

❧EPILOGUE❧

"THERE'S NO PLACE LIKE HOME . . ."

As I sat here at the computer this morning putting the finishing touches on my book, I was worried about one of my hives. I knew it was overcrowded and ready to swarm. (The bees will create a new queen when there's not enough space in the hive. Then thousands of bees leave the hive with the queen and look for a new home.) The bees had attempted to swarm last weekend but the queen did not follow. It was an amazing sight. First, thousands of bees were crawling all over the hive. Then, they flew over the house. It looked and sounded like something out of an Alfred Hitchcock movie. I ran inside to get my camera. I took many pictures but my lens was not powerful enough to capture the experience on film. Eventually, they moved from the top of the house toward the backyard. I was right in their path. I was very frightened. I ran into the house as they flew by me in search of a home. I did not get stung.

❧ ❧ ❧

FIRST, THOUSANDS OF BEES WERE CRAWLING ALL OVER THE HIVE. THEN, THEY FLEW OVER THE HOUSE. IT LOOKED AND SOUNDED LIKE SOMETHING OUT OF AN ALFRED HITCHCOCK MOVIE.

❧ ❧ ❧

My 16 year old son ran upstairs and said, "Mom, what's happening?" I explained that the bees from one of the hives had swarmed to a nearby tree. They were buzzing around in mid-air. What a sight to see, a free-for-all! I called George Imrie, a master beekeeper in my area. He had the greatest message on his machine: "This is honeybee swarm season! If you're calling because you have a swarm, I WANT THE BEES! I check my messages every hour. Please leave your name and number and I WILL call you back."

By the time he returned my call, the bees had gone back to their hive and were crawling all over the outside. I told him that I didn't understand what was happening. He explained that the queen did not follow the scout bees. "Can you come over anyway and take away the swarm?," I asked, naively. "Everything is over for today," he said. "There's nothing else you can do. They'll probably try it again soon."

I was fascinated with the whole event, but I kept a watchful eye on the colony all week. I was both exhilarated by the experience and yet fearful. As you have no doubt figured out by now, I am a novice beekeeper who loves helping people with apitherapy. I have felt inadequate to manage my own hives. My main concern has been that the hives would swarm to my neighbors' yards and somehow I would be prevented from doing my healing work.

I made many calls this week to try and find an experienced beekeeper who would take me under his wing. I was unsuccessful. Out of sheer desperation this afternoon, when I saw the hive beginning to swarm again, I asked God for help. "You've got to help me with this," I prayed. "I don't know what to do! These bees need a new home. Please send someone who can help me."

Five minutes later I glanced out the window and the bees were gone. They were no longer climbing all over the front of the hive. "Oh, my God," I thought. "They've already swarmed." I ran outside looking for them. There they were up in my pine tree, 30 feet above the ground. They were hanging from a branch like a bunch of grapes. I was excited. I called my friend Greg Ferris. Thank God he was home. He told me that I had nothing to worry about. "They'll be gone in a day or two. Out here in the country, we shoot them down, but in Bethesda that would probably not be very appropriate."

We discussed the possibility that I could catch the swarm myself. I told him I had some extra hive bodies in the basement. He asked if I had any "drawn comb," frames that still had comb on them after the honey had been extracted. I told him that I thought I might have some downstairs. "We'll make a beekeeper out of you yet!" he chuckled. And I replied, "Ten or fifteen years from now I'll probably remind you about the time you helped me catch my first swarm."

I was so proud of myself as I single handedly prepared a new home for my swarming bees. I felt invigorated and empowered. This was quite a change from the feelings of inadequacy that I had experienced earlier in the day. I was so excited that I started writing this epilogue in my head as I gathered my equipment together. "What a great adventure this has been," I thought to myself.

And what a year it has been! To think, just a year ago, I was sitting in my backyard with nothing to do. I felt like I had no reason to be in Bethesda. There was nothing holding me here. And now, I have every reason to be in Bethesda.

I carried my equipment outside, getting a little out of breath as a walked up the basement steps. The sky was blue and the clouds were rolling by. And suddenly I looked up and I noticed the swarm was gone! I was stunned and surprised. I stood there holding the white hive body as time stood still . . .

And then a line from the Wizard of Oz kept repeating itself over and over again in my mind:

"There's no place like home, there's no place like home . . ."

The bees have found a new home and so have I. I am at home in Bethesda. I am at home in myself. It is not a coincidence that the very name Bethesda brings to mind Biblical references. Bethesda is a Hebrew word for "House of Mercy." Bethesda was a pool where Jesus healed an invalid and gave him the power to walk. Some say that Bethesda was the name of a Jewish angel who healed people at the edge of a pool. Others claim that Bethesda is a place in Israel where the Ten Commandments are hidden.

In any case, Bethesda has become a very wonderful place for me. The tradition of healing continues in Bethesda. It is a place to heal myself and others. Just as Lonny is starting to walk again, I, too, am taking steps towards my own healing.

I have recently come to understand that Bethesda is a state of mind. I know now, that I could go anywhere and BEE IN BALANCE. Everything has the possibility of turning into its opposite. The starpoint within us will guide us home.

Amber Rose

CONSULTATIONS WITH THE AUTHOR

Personalized consultations are available from the author by phone and in person. Consultations are intended for those who have followed the suggestions outlined in this book and are having difficulty determining the best approach to Bee Venom Therapy, such as knowing what element is out of balance and where to sting. Consultations need to be arranged in advance by calling Amber Rose at (301) 530-0472 during regular business hours. The fee for these consultations is $100/hour or $50/half hour. It is recommended that you fill out the case history form at the end of the book and send it to the author before arranging the consultation, as this will reduce your expenses.

SOLICITATION OF ANECDOTES & IDEAS

The author welcomes all anecdotes and ideas for her companion volume to Bee in Balance, currently titled "The Jade Bee and Other Stories." Please send your stories and comments to:

Amber Rose, L.Ac., L.C.S.W.
Starpoint Enterprises, Ltd.
5419 Roosevelt Street
Bethesda, MD 20817

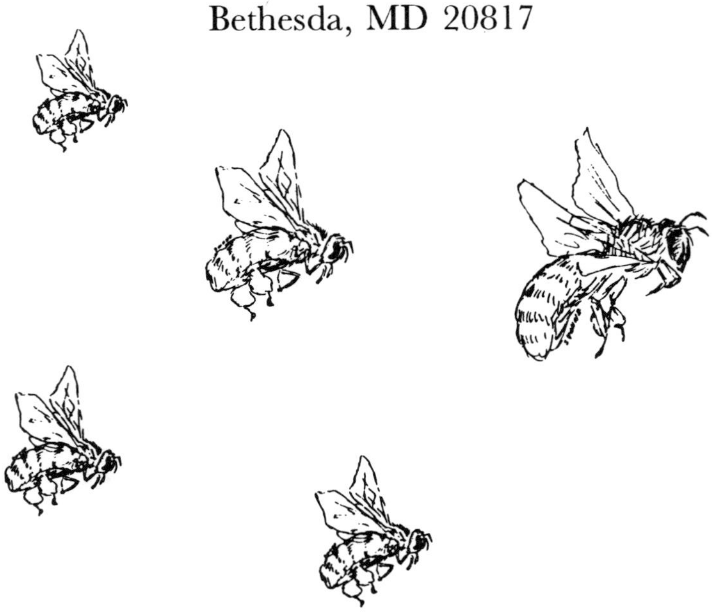

APPENDICES

APPENDIX I

GLOSSARY

AGGRESSIVE ENERGY (AE) It is an invasive energy that knocks us off balance. It is harmful energy that is going in the wrong direction. It is energy that stagnates and then moves across the K'o cycle; a metaphor for this would be that the grandmother is sick and turns on the grandchild. Aggressive Energy is one step beyond reasonable control. It is very destructive and deep seated. The danger is to the yin organs: the liver, the heart, the heart protector, the spleen, the lungs and the kidneys. AE can be triggered by an acute or devastating trauma or a chronic condition, i.e., pain or illness.

CAUSATIVE FACTOR (CF) This is the element or the official that was first knocked off balance in childhood and was unable to bounce back. This is the weakest link in the chain. This is the deepest injury. This is where we shine and where we struggle. This is the element or the pathway that will affect all the others. Treating this pathway will be like bringing water to a desert, it will change everything. This is not necessarily the pathway or element that has the most symptoms. Diagnosing the CF is based on the color on the face around the eyes, the sound of the voice, the odor, and the emotion which is most out of balance. The selection of the element and pathways out of balance described in this book is not necessarily the CF.

CH'I (QI) This is the energy or life force that flows through the meridians. The ultimate cause of disease is an imbalance in the *Ch'i.*

CHINESE CLOCK During the 24 hours in a day there is a circulation of energy from the heart pathway to the spleen pathway. Since there are 12 meridians, each meridian has a peak time for two hours (See horary points for the time of day for each pathway). The order in which the *Ch'i* flows through the clock is important for Oriental diagnosis and treatment. (See Horary). It is important when calculating time to use "sun time" instead of "daylight savings" time.

COMMAND POINTS These are points that are found from the elbow crease to the finger tips and the knee crease to the toes. These are points by which we command the whole meridian at once. We're saying, "Do this."

KINDS OF COMMAND POINTS

Tonification points	Horary points
Sedation Points	Junction points
Source points	Element points

ELEMENT POINTS There is a point on every pathway that corresponds to each element. Each pathway contains one point for each of the five elements; i.e., there is a wood, fire, earth, metal and water point on each pathway.

ENTRY POINTS The *Ch'i* energy enters the meridian at this point. This is usually, but not always, the first point on the pathway. The energy entering at this point has just left the exit point of the previous meridian. For the order of the flow of energy (See Chinese Clock or Horary).

ENTRY/EXIT BLOCK Each pathway begins with an entry point and flows toward an exit point. These points are like gateways. They can be rusted shut or open. This would be an entry/exit block. It can be easily corrected by treating the entry and exit points on one pathway and perhaps the entry and exit points on the pathway which follows it according to the Chinese Clock (See Chinese Clock). If you are having symptoms at the same time every day you probably have an entry/exit block. You will need to flush out the pathway. For example, the time of day that goes with the liver pathway is 1 a.m.—3 a.m. If you are consistently waking up in the middle of the night at this time, it means you have an entry/exit block on the liver. You would need to treat LV-1 and LV-13 and 14 (the liver has two exit points). But if you are waking up at 3:15 a.m., that is in the lung time, so in this case you might want to treat the liver exit points and the entry point on the lungs, L-1.

Here are the main indications that you probably need to use entry/exit points:

✗ When two or more consecutive pathways are having trouble. In this case consecutive means according to the Chinese Clock. This means that you would continue to have symptoms at the same time almost every day.

✗ When the patient is doing well and then all of a sudden the old symptoms come back.

✗ You have tried everything and nothing seems to be working and the patient feels discouraged.

✗ If you do a treatment and you get no response.

✗ Scars can often block a pathway. Do the closest entry/exit points.

EXIT POINTS These are the point where the energy exits from a pathway. This is usually, but not always, the last point on the pathway (See entry points and entry/exit blocks).

EXTERNAL DRAGONS A condition where the person makes very little eye contact. It's hard to connect with this person. This is often caused by something that comes at you from the outside such as food poisoning, AIDS, polio, encephalitis, a car accident, a rape, sexual or physical abuse, a trauma, a fall, being exposed to the elements for too long (wind, heat, fire, dampness, humidity, dryness, and cold). The points used to correct this condition are: Governor Vessel 20, Bladder 11 (bilateral), Bladder 23 (bilateral) and Bladder 61 (bilateral).

FIRST AID POINTS These points are only used to get the patient through an acute situation. They are not used for mild discomfort or a chronic situation. This is not a five element treatment. It is based on symptoms rather than an oriental diagnosis. It may clear the symptoms more quickly, but the results may not be permanent.

FORBIDDEN POINTS Points which are forbidden to sting; these are points which are forbidden to treat with moxa, an herb used to apply heat to the point. These are points which you may use for acupressure, but never sting them with a bee. These points are marked with an **F**.

GOVERNOR VESSEL (DU MO) This meridian runs up the back of the spine. It is part of the eight extra meridians and is not ruled by the five elements. It is the most yang meridian of the body.

HEALING CRISIS Somewhere between the first and the fifth bee sting treatment you may notice some flu-like symptoms or some nausea. You may feel tired and achy, and you may not want to get out of bed or go through your usual daily routine. Don't despair. This will not last very long, maybe one or two days, although it does vary from person to person. It is a good sign that toxins are leaving your system and being flushed out through the bloodstream. So, don't worry, the healing crisis will not last forever. You have to push through it. You can cut down on your number of stings for a treatment or two, but then you can build back up again. The most important thing to remember is that this is normal and nothing to worry about. When you are not feeling well, you may be tempted to give up, but I urge you to continue if you can. Remember "this too shall pass."

HOME ELEMENT POINT There is a point on every pathway that the same element as the pathway, i.e., a wood point on a wood pathway or a fire point on a fire pathway. When used during the right time of day or the right season, it is considered a horary point (See Horary Point).

HORARY POINT This is the pathway's home element point. An example of this would be a fire point on a fire pathway or a wood point on a wood pathway. A horary point is only effective as a horary treatment during either the two hour segment of the day, when the pathway is at its peak, or during the season with which its associated. This point calls up the nature of the element at the right time of day. So if you do a fire point on a fire pathway at the fire time of day, then you are getting triple the value. And if you do it in the right season, then you get four times the value. You can do just a seasonal horary treatment. This would be doing a fire point on a fire pathway at the right time of year, but not at the right time of day. As another example, let's say it is springtime and you want to strengthen the liver pathway. You know that you want to use a horary point to do this, but you don't want to stay up until 1 a.m. So you do a seasonal horary treatment. You treat the wood point on the liver but you don't focus on what time of day it is.

By using the horary point on the patient you can revitalize the whole person. Here is a list of all the horary points:

11pm—1am	WOOD/GB-41
1am—3am	WOOD/LV-1
3am—5am	METAL/L-8
5am—7am	METAL/CO-1
7am—9am	EARTH/ST-36
9am—11am	EARTH/SP-3
11am—1pm	FIRE/H-8
1pm—3pm	FIRE/SI-5
3pm—5pm	WATER/BL-66
5pm—7pm	WATER/K-10
7pm—9pm	FIRE/HP-8
9pm—11pm	FIRE/TH-6

HUSBAND/WIFE IMBALANCE A Husband and Wife Imbalance occurs when the pulse picture reflects a reversal in the natural order, in which the Husband (the left hand) is weaker than the Wife (the right hand). This is a condition which requires a trained acupuncturist to diagnose correctly.

INTERNAL DRAGONS A condition where the person does not make good eye contact. They feel controlled by their emotions. They may feel stuck in an emotion like anger, grief, joy, worry, or fear. Their life feels very chaotic and their symptoms are very persistent. This condition is treated by seven points: the master point below Conception Vessel 15, Stomach 25 (bilateral), Stomach 32 (bilateral), and Stomach 41 (bilateral).

JUNCTION POINT A junction point joins the two paired meridians (meridians in the same element constitute a pair; the four fire meridians constitute two pairs), so the yin and yang energy can be balanced. The junction point is a gateway that reconnects the two pathways. Be sure to work on all the pathways that go with each element. For example, if you just work on the liver and not the gall bladder, the gall bladder may get jealous and therefore produce symptoms.

K'O CYCLE This is a control cycle. The energy skips a generation. The grandmother controls the grandchild. Wood is the mother of fire. Fire is the mother of earth, therefore, wood is the grandmother of earth. So, wood controls earth, earth controls water, water controls fire, fire controls metal, and metal controls wood. If this check system gets out of control, it becomes a destructive cycle. This is called Aggressive Energy.

LAW OF LEAST ACTION The less treatment that is done, the more effective it becomes. There is more of an impact with a single message. When you over-treat a patient, you can lose some ground. It is like over-watering a plant.

PULSES An acupuncturist takes pulses very differently than a Western doctor. The acupuncture practitioner reads six pulses on each wrist. What is being felt is the *Ch'i* energy in each organ and/or pathway. They are feeling for the quality of the pulse, instead of counting the number of beats, as does a Western doctor.

SEDATE Sedation disperses excess energy, allowing the point to relax; like turning off the car motor, or at least taking one's foot off the accelerator. This is done when there is excess energy on that pathway. Specific acupuncture techniques can be used to sedate acupuncture points; this is usually done by leaving acupuncture needles in the point for an extended period. Since bee stings tonify, it is thought that bee stings cannot be used to sedate.

SEDATION POINT A sedation point is the child point on that pathway. For example, fire is the child of wood. A sedation point on the wood pathway would be the fire point on the wood pathway. The sedation point will sedate the pathway or allow it to relax.

SHEN CYCLE The shen cycle follows the order of the seasons: spring (wood), summer (fire), late summer (earth), autumn or fall (metal) and winter (water). The elements are inseparable; they are involved in a continuous dance of energy. There is no beginning and no end; you cannot have one without the other. Each element gives birth to the next element on the cycle.

SOURCE POINT This point will allow you to bring the most perfect energy to that meridian or pathway. Source points are considered to be the safest points on the body. They bring exactly what is needed. A source point is a reservoir of perfect energy.

SPECIAL POINTS These are points that are used to treat chronic conditions. Points used in this way are not part of Five Element Acupuncture, but are being used to treat symptoms only. They may be effective in the short-run, but they do not get down to the root cause.

SPIRIT OF THE POINT This refers to the meaning of the point based on the name of that point. Gate of Hope (LV—14), for example, is a good point when someone feels hopeless.

TONIFY This means to strengthen or add energy to a point; like turning over the ignition on your car. Bee stings are a potent way to tonify a pathway or a point.

TONIFICATION POINT A tonification point is the mother point on that pathway. For example, wood is the mother of fire. Therefore, the wood point on a fire pathway will be the tonification point. When treated this point will stimulate the person. It would be like turning the ignition on in the car.

WINDOWS OF THE SKY There are 11 Windows of the Sky. Most of them are on the neck or close to it. A Window is indicated when the person really wants a breakthrough. One has to be ready. Your patient will ask you for it, and even beg for it. The person may say, "I really want to see what happened in my childhood," "I'm at the end of my rope, I have to break through all this soon!" or "I feel cut off from the neck down." In general, when any of us goes through a major trauma in childhood, we may shut down. In this case we may close down our Windows. Tonifying a Window will help the person to open up more. Windows bring the body, mind and spirit together.

APPENDIX II
READING LIST
ABOUT BEES

BEEKEEPING AND HONEYBEE PRODUCTS

Brown, Royden. Bee Hive Product Bible. New York: Avery Publishing Group, Inc., 1993.

Dadant & Sons (editors). The Hive and the Honeybee. Illinois: Dadant and Sons, revised edition 1975.

Kelley, Walter T. How to Keep Bees and Sell Honey. Kentucky: 1993 (13th edition).

Sammataro, Diana, and Alphonse Avitabile. The Beekeeper's Handbook. New York: Collier Books, 1986.

Hubbell, Sue. A Country Year, Living the Questions. New York: Harper and Row, 1983.

BEE VENOM THERAPY

Beck, Bodog, M.D. Bee Venom Therapy. New York: D. Appleton Century Co., 1935.

Lloyd, James. God's Answer to Suffering: Bee Venom Therapy Techniques. To be completed in 1994.

Malone, Fred. Bees Don't Get Arthritis. New York: E.P Dutton, 1979.

Mraz, Charles. Health and the Honeybee. Burlington, VT: Queen City Publishing, 1994.

Simics, Michael. Bee Venom: Exploring the Healing Power. Alberta, Canada: Apitronic Services, 1994.

Wagner, Pat. How Well Are You Willing to Bee? To be completed in 1994.

ABOUT HEALING

ACUPUNCTURE

Beinfield, Harriet, R.Ac., and Efrem Korngold, L.Ac., O.M.D. Between Heaven and Earth. New York: Ballantine Books, 1991.

Connelly, Dianne. Traditional Acupuncture: The Law of the Five Elements. Columbia, MD: The Center for Traditional Acupuncture, Inc. (5th edition) 1992.

Connelly, Dianne. All Sickness is Homesickness. Columbia, MD: The Traditional Acupuncture Institute, 1993.

Ellis, Andrew, and Nigel Wiseman, and Ken Boss. Fundamentals of Chinese Acupuncture. Massachusetts: Paradigm Publications, 1991.

Kaptchuk, Ted. The Web That Has No Weaver. New York: Congdon and Weed, 1992.

McGarey, William A. Acupuncture and Body Energies. Arizona: Gabriel Press, 1974.

Mann, Felix, M.B. Acupuncture: The Ancient Chinese Art of Healing and How it Works Scientifically. New York: Vintage Books, 1973.

O'Connor, John, and Dan Bensky. Acupuncture, A Comprehensive Text. Seattle: Eastland Press, 1981.

Seem, Mark, Ph.D. Acupuncture Energetics. Vermont: Healing Arts Press, 1987.

Worsley, J.R. Is Acupuncture for You? New York: Harper and Row, 1973.

BACH FLOWER REMEDIES

Bach, Edward, M.D., and F.J. Wheeler. The Bach Flower Remedies. New Caanan, CT: Keats, 1979.

Kaslof, Leslie J. The Bach Remedies: A Self-Help Guide. New Caanan, CT: Keats, 1988.

Scheffer, Mechtild. Bach Flower Therapy. Rochester, VT: Inner Traditions, 1987.

BODYWORK

Barlow, Wilfred. The Alexander Technique. New York: Alfred A. Knopf, 1991.

Byers, Dwight. Better Health with Foot Reflexology. Florida: Ingham Publishing, 1987.

Feldenkrais, Moshe. Awareness through Movement: Health Exercises for Personal Growth. New York: Harper and Row, 1972.

Gach, Michael, R. Acupressure's Potent Points. New York: Bantam Books, 1990.

Gach, Michael, R. Acu-Yoga. Tokyo and New York: Bantam Books, 1990.

Krieger, Dolores. Living the Therapeutic Touch: Healing as a Lifestyle. Illinois: Quest Books, 1988.

Lidell, Lucinda. The Book of Massage. New York: Fireside, 1984.

Prudden, Bonnie. Myotherapy. New York: Ballantine Books, 1985.

Stone, Randolph. Polarity Therapy: The Complete and Collected Works. Vol. 1 and 2. CA: CRCS Publications, 1987.

CHELATION THERAPY

Trowbridge, John P., M.D. and Morton Walker, D.P.M. Chelation Therapy, the Healing Powers. Stamford, CT: New Way of Life, Inc., 1988.

Walker, Morton, D.P.M. The Chelation Way. Garden City Park, NY: Avery Publishing Group, Inc., 1990.

CHIROPRACTIC

Palmer, Daniel, David. The Chiropractor's Adjuster. Davenport, IA: Palmer College Press, 1992.

Wilk, Chester. Chiropractic Speaks Out. Chicago: Wilk Publishing Co., 1975.

EMOTIONAL/SPIRITUAL HEALING

Beattie, Melody. Codependent No More. New York: Harper and Row, Publishers, Inc., 1987.

Beattie, Melody. The Language of Letting Go. San Francisco: Harper and Row, Publishers, 1990.

Campanella, Roy. It's Good to Be Alive. Boston: Little, Brown and Co., 1959.

Hay, Louise. You Can Heal Your Life. Santa Monica, CA: Hay House, 1989.

Redfield, James. The Celestine Prophecy, An Adventure. New York: Warner Books, Inc., 1994.

Siegel, Bernie S., M.D. Peace, Love and Healing. New York: Harper Perrenial, 1990.

Siegel, Bernie S., M.D. Love, Medicine and Miracles. New York: Harper and Row, 1988.

FOLK MEDICINE

Jarvis, D.C., M.D. Vermont Folk Medicine. New York: Henry Holt and Co., 1958.

Jarvis, D.C., M.D. Arthritis and Folk Medicine. New York: Fawcett Crest Books, 1960.

HERBS

Black, Dean. Regeneration! China's Ancient Gift to the Modern Quest for Health. Utah: Tapestry Press (Bioresearch Foundation), 1988. (1-800-333-4290)

Kloss, Jethro. Back to Eden. California: Back to Eden Books, 1939.

HOMEOPATHY

Lockie, Andrew. The Family Guide to Homeopathy: Symptoms and Natural Solutions. New York: Prentice Hall Press, 1993.

Ullman, Dana. Discovering Homeopathy: Your Introduction to the Science and Art of Homeopathic Medicine. Berkeley, CA.: North Atlantic Books, 1991.

NATUROPHY

Murray, Michael, N.D. and Joseph Pizzorno, N.D. A Textbook of Natural Medicine, Vol 1 & 2. Seattle: John Bastyr College Publications, 1989.

Murray, Michael, N.D. and Joseph Pizzorno, N.D. Encyclopedia of Natural Medicine. Rocklin, CA: Prima Publishing, 1991.

NUTRITION

Balch, James F., M.D. and Phyllis A. Balch, C.N.C. Prescription for Nutritional Healing. New York: Avery Publishing Group, Inc., 1990.

Brody, Jane. Jane Brody's Nutrition Book. New York: Bantam Books, 1982.

Beasley, Joseph D.,M.D. and Susan Knightly. Food for Recovery. New York: Crown Trade Paperbacks, 1994.

Berger, Stuart M., M.D. How To Be Your Own Nutritionist. New York: Avon Books, 1987.

Bieler, Henry G., M.D. Food is Your Best Medicine. New York: Ballantine Books, 1982.

Colbin, Annemarie. Food and Healing. New York: Ballantine Books, 1986.

Mindell, Earl, R.Ph., Ph.D. Earl Mindell's Food as Medicine. New York: Simon and Schuster, 1994.

Quillin, Patrick, Ph.D., R.D. Healing Nutrients. New York: Vintage Books, 1989.

Wade, Carlson. Health from the Hive. Connecticut: Keats Publishing, Inc., 1992.

OSTEOPATHY

Trowbridge, Carol. Andrew Taylor Still—1828-1917. Kirksville, MO: Thomas Jefferson University Press, 1991.

PREVENTIVE MEDICINE

Fox, Arnold, M.D. and Barry Fox, Ph.D. Immune for Life. California: Prima Publishing, 1990.

Giller, Robert M., M.D. and Kathy Matthew. Natural Prescriptions. New York: Carol Southern Books, 1994.

Nyoiti, Sakurazawa. You are All Sanpaku. New York: Award Books, 1970.

ABOUT DISEASES AND AILMENTS

ALLERGIES

Randolph, Theron G., M.D., and Ralph W. Moss, Ph.D. An Alternative Approach to Allergies. New York: Harper and Row, 1980, Bantam, 1982.

AMALGAMS

Huggins, Hal A., D.D.S., M.S. It's All in Your Head: The Link Between Mercury Amalgams and Illness. New York: Avery Publishing Group, Inc., 1993.

CANDIDA (YEAST SENSITIVITY)

Crook, William, M.D. The Yeast Connection. New York: Vintage, 1986.

Trowbridge, John Parks and Morton Walker, D.P.M. The Yeast Syndrome. New York: Bantam Books, 1986.

Gates, Donna. The Body Ecology Diet. Atlanta: B.E.D. Publishing, 1993.

MULTIPLE SCLEROSIS

Graham, Judy. Multiple Sclerosis: A Self Help Guide to Its Management. Vermont: Healing Arts Press, 1989.

Soll, Robert W., M.D. MS: Something Can Be Done and You Can Do It! Chicago: Contemporary Books, 1984.

ABOUT RELAXING!

MEDITATION

Benson, Herbert. The Relaxation Response. New York: Morrow, 1975.

Borysenko, Joan. Minding the Body, Mending the Mind. New York: Bantam Books, 1988.

Goleman, Daniel. The Meditative Mind. Los Angeles: Jeremy P. Tarcher, Inc., 1988.

Kabat-Zinn, Jon, Ph.D. Full Catastrophe Living. New York: Dell Publishing, 1990.

Ram Dass, Baba. Be Here Now. New York: Crown, 1971.

Ram Dass, Baba. The Only Dance There Is. New York: Anchor/Doubleday, 1974.

Roth, Robert. Transcendental Meditation. New York: Donald I. Fine, Inc., 1988.

YOGA

Iyengar, B.K.S. Light on Yoga, Revised edition. New York: Schocken Books, 1977.

Vishnudevananda, Swami. The Complete Illustrated Book of Yoga. New York: Harmony Books, 1980.

VIDEO TAPES AVAILABLE FROM THE AMERICAN APITHERAPY SOCIETY (AAS)

Physician, Heal Thyself; The Charles Mraz Story. $50

AAS 1993 Tour of China. $50

"I Want to Tell the World," available from the New Hampshire State Beekeeping Association and can be ordered from Mike Bayco, 69 Bean Road, Merrimack, NH 03054 (603) 424-5477. $15

IMPORTANT NAMES AND ADDRESSES

BEES BY MAIL	GREG FERRIS Rt. No. 1 Box 460-H Indian Head, MD 20640 800-787-HONY
APITHERAPY AND MS, ARTHRITIS, ETC., LECTURES, & GUIDES	PAT WAGNER 5419 Lucy Drive Waldorf, MD 20601 301-843-8350 "HOW WELL ARE YOU WILLING TO BEE?"
"BEE—ACUPUNCTURE" FOR MS, ARTHRITIS, ETC., EDUCATIONAL CONSULTATIONS (FACE TO FACE AND PHONE) LECTURES, SEMINARS; PLEASE SEND ANECDOTES FOR NEXT BOOK.	AMBER ROSE 5419 Roosevelt St. Bethesda, MD 20817 301-530-0472
APITHERAPY FOR MS, ARTHRITIS, ETC., AND BEE VENOM SOLUTION	CHARLES MRAZ Box 127 Middlebury, VT 05753 802-388-2995 "HEALTH AND THE HONEYBEE" is available from: QUEEN CITY PUBLISHING c/o Michelle Mraz-Kurker 1123 Pine Street Burlington, VT 05401
CERTIFICATION PROGRAM, ATTORNEY, APITHERAPY, BVT BOOK	JIM LLYOD 1515 E. 71 St., Suite 200 Tulsa, OK 74136 918-492-2161 (office)

Certification program for apitherapy	CONTACT PERSON: DIANE MCGUIRE Rodgers State College Claremore, OK 74017 918-341-7510 This is a six month certification course taught by Jim Lloyd given twice a year, 1 evening/week for 2 hrs. A correspondence course is also available. Weekend/weeklong certification programs are planned.
Information packets Membership, Research and data collection	AMERICAN APITHERAPY ASSOCIATION (AAS) P.O. Box 54, Rt.12 Hartland Four Corners, VT 05049 800-823-3460
Adverse reactions	TH. CHERBULIEZ 1209 Post Rd. Scarsdale, NY 10583-2023 Tel/Fax: 914-723-0920
Whole dried bee venom, bee venom solution, bee venom collection devices and technology, and books and booklets on bee venom and its technology	MICHAEL SIMICS Apitronic Services 204 1331 15th Ave. S.W. Calgary, Alberta T3COX8, Canada Tel/Fax: 403-541-1877
Legal Assistance Regarding the Problems of Alternative Health Care Providers	ALAN DUMOFF Law Office of Alan Dumoff 3102 Blueford Road Kensington, MD 20895 301-949-9053

SUNRIDER HERBS	DAVID TOWNSEND 5501 Glenridge Drive Apt. #514 Atlanta, Georgia 30342 404-303-7777
EAST COAST POLLEN	ANDY FILANGERI 269 S. Mountain Rd. Gardiner, N.Y. 12525
MEBO AND BURN THERAPY	PROF. HARRY GAYNOR National Burn Victim Foundation 32 Scotland Rd. Orange, NJ 07050 201-676-7700
MENTAL HEALTH AND LIFESTYLE COUNSELOR TELEPHONE CONSULTATIONS	DR. MYRNA ALEXANDER 3850 South 9th Road Arlington, VA 22204 703-979-5159
WELLNESS CONSULTANT VIBRATIONAL MEDICINE TELEPHONE CONSULTATIONS, LECTURES AND SEMINARS	ALICIA FOSTER, M.S. LIFESONG Sciences 3900 Juan Tabot Blvd. N.E. Suite 263A Albequerque, NM 87111 505-298-1689

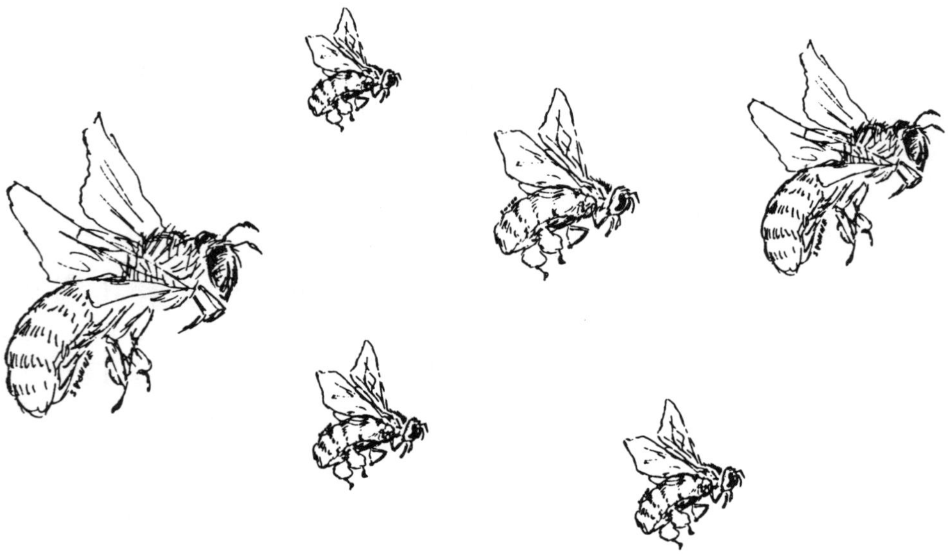

APPENDIX III

For more detailed information, see Michael Simics' book, Bee Venom: Exploring the Healing Power. Alberta, Canada: Apitronic Services, 1994. My thanks to Michael for his assistance in compiling the following information:

The Component parts in Honeybee Venom:

There are 76 different components in bee venom, but not all of these components are consistently present in every bee's venom. There are six primary components which are thought to provide the major therapeutic benefits of BVT.

Hyaluronidase:

Physiological Properties: loosens the glue which connects cells, making the tissue more permeable. Healing substances have greater access to the cells; the elimination of toxic substances also becomes easier.

Phospholipase A1 & A2:

Physiological properties: contained in all venoms, it is an emulsifier which acts to detoxify the cells.

Apamin:

Physiological Properties: assists damaged nerve receptors by specifically enhancing critical aspects of nerve transmission.

Melittin:

Physiological Properties: Melittin attacks certain cell walls, creating the "sting." It has bacteriocidal and other healing properties. While it causes the histamine reaction which causes swelling and inflammation, it has strong anti-inflammatory effects.

Histamine:

Physiological Properties: produces signs of inflammation, well known to allergic suffers who get relief from their symptoms using anti-histamines.

Mast Cell Degranulating Peptide:

Physiological Properties: another agent which leads to the release of histamine. It has positive effects on neurochemistry. It may produce a feeling of mental alertness and improved concentration.

The following compounds also exist in some bee venom and are also known to have beneficial effects:

"Compound X":

Physiological Properties: appears to potentiate the effectiveness of other compounds in the venom.

Dopamine:

Physiological Properties: A neurotransmitter that increases motor activity.

Norepinephrine:

Physiological Properties: a neurotransmitter that mediates the "fight or flight" response.

Adolapin:

Physiological Properties: an anti-inflammatory agent which produces an analgesic effect.

Anecdotal Reports regarding BVT in Clinical Practice

Neurological:
- multiple sclerosis
- chronic low back pain
- sciatica
- lumbago
- analgesia

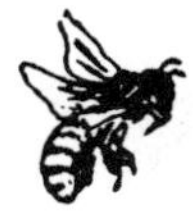

Rheumatological:
- rheumatoid and traumatic arthritis
- juvenile rheumatoid arthritis
- osteoarthritis
- bursitis (shoulder, knee)
- myalgias (muscle spasms/pains)
- ankylyosing spondylitis deformans
- polyarteritis deformans
- psoriatic arthritis
- tennis elbow
- Schlermann's disease

Immune system:
- immune augmentation
- some cancers (studies in progress)
- lupus

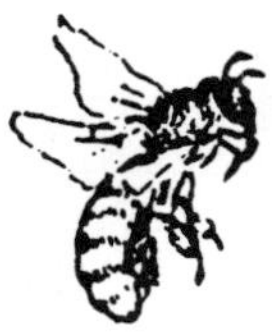
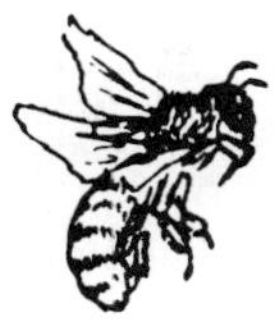

Dermatological:
- eczema
- psoriasis
- sclerolysis
- scleroderma
- topical ulcers
- degranulating wounds
- corns

Cardiovascular/Respiratory:
- high blood pressure
- peripheral vascular diseases

- arrhythmias
- atherosclerosis
- diabetic neuropathy
- emphysema
- asthma

Sense Organs:
- improves hearing and eyesight

Healing/Prevention:
- stimulates healing of bones, wounds, lesions, and scars
- stimulates/prevents colds and flu-like illnesses

Psych/Endocrine:
- decreased blood sugar
- depression; mood swings
- PMS; menstrual cramps, regular periods
- female fertility and increased sperm count

Viral:
- meningitis
- herpes
- shingles
- warts

Components of Bee Pollen, the "Most Perfect Food" available:

Vitamins:
Vitamins A, B1, B2, B3, B6, Pantothenic acid, Biotin, B12, folic acid, choline, inositol; Vitamins C, D, E, and rutin.

Minerals:
calcium, phosphorous, zinc, silicon, molybden, boron, titanium, potassium, sulfur, sodium, chlorine, magnesium, iron, manganese, copper, iodine.

Protein/Amino Acids:
alanine, aspartic acid, glutamic acid, tryptophan, isoleucine, leucine, lysine, methionine, phenylalanine, threonine, valine, histidine, arginine, cystine, tyrosine, hydroxyproline, proline, serine.

Enzymes:
amylase, diastase, saccharase, pectase, phosphatase, catalase, diaphorase, cozymase, cytochrome systems, lactic dehydrogenase, succinic dehydrogenase, 24 oxidoreductases, 21 transferases, 33 hydrolases, 11 lyases, 5 isomerases, pepsin, trypsin.

Others:
nucleic acids, flavonoids, terpenes, nucleosides, auxins, fructose, glucose, brassins, gibberellins, kinins, vernine, guanine, xanthine, hypoxanthine, nuclein, amines, lecithin, xanthophylls, crocetin, zeaxanthin, lycopene, hexodecanal, alpha-amino-butyric-acid, monoglycerides, diglycerides, triglycerides, pentosans.

Components of Propolis ("Russian Penicillin"):

According to Royden Brown in his book, "Bee Hive Product Bible," propolis is 55% resinous compounds and balsam, 30% beeswax, 10% ethereal and aromatic oils, and 5% pollen.

It also includes: flavonols, chrysin, galangin, vanillin, pinocembrin, caffeic acid, cinnamic acid, tetochrysin, cinnamyl alcohol, and ferulic acid.

Research shows that propolis is antifungal, antiviral, antibacterial, antiseptic, antibiotic, anti-inflammatory, as well as an anesthetic. There have been anecdotal reports that propolis has been helpful for toothaches, gum problems, asthma, heartburn, and skin conditions.

Components of Royal Jelly:

As described by Carlson Wade in his book, "Health from the Hive," royal jelly contains all the B vitamins, including a large concentration of B-5 and B-6. It also includes: pure acetylcholine, vitamin A, C, D, and E, minerals, hormones, enzymes, and 18 amino acids. Royal jelly is 66% water, 12.5% protein, 12.5% carbohydrates, 5% fat and 4% unknown materials.

Royal jelly has antibacterial and antibiotic components. Royal jelly is known to help liver disease, asthma, insomnia, pancreatitis, kidney disease, stomach ulcers, bone fractures, and skin disorders. It also helps the immune system.

Royal jelly spoils easily and needs to be refrigerated or mixed with honey.

There are anecdotal reports that royal jelly increases energy in general and sexual energy. It is also helpful in cases of infertility. It also reduces blood pressure, decreases triglyceride levels and stimulates appetite.

Components of Raw Honey:

Royden Brown describes raw honey as having Vitamin A, all the vitamin B's, as well as C, D, E, and K. It also contains the following minerals: potassium, iodine, calcium, phosphorous, iron, chlorine, copper, sodium, and manganese.

One of the most important things about raw honey is that it hasn't been heated and therefore it still has live enzymes. Honey also has proteins, organic acids, carbohydrates and antibiotic qualities. Honey also contains dextrose, levulose, and dextrose.

Raw honey is especially good internally for allergies, asthma, bronchitis, sinusitis. Apple cider vinegar and honey mixed with warm water is good for colds. Externally, raw honey is good for burns, wounds, and bedsores because it is a topical antibiotic. Honey is also helpful for athlete's foot since it has antifungal properties. If you mix honey and warm water, it makes a good eye wash for conjunctivitis. There have also been reports that cataracts have been successfully treated by placing a drop of raw honey in the eye at bedtime.

APPENDIX IV

FORMS

ASSUMPTION OF LIABILITY

TO WHOM IT MAY CONCERN:

I, ______________________________, do hereby state that it is with my complete consent and it is my firm desire to be stung by honeybees at the home of ________________. No promises or guarantees have been made to me with regard to what the honeybee stings may or may not do to alter my present health status. Furthermore, I understand that any health condition I have may be MADE WORSE by being stung by honeybees. Nevertheless, IT IS my firm desire to be stung by said honeybees.

I understand that there are four types of reactions that are possible from being stung by honeybees: Generalized Immediate, Localized Immediate, Generalized Delayed, and Localized Delayed. It has been explained to me that Anaphylactic Shock falls into the category of Generalized Immediate, and that it might result in my death. I agree not to hold Amber Rose responsible for any undesirable effect which may result from said honeybee stings given to me at her home.

Address________________ Signed______________________

City___________________ Dated_______________________

St. and Zip____________ Witness_____________________

Home Phone_____________

Work Phone_____________

CASE HISTORY

NAME ____

ADDRESS ____

CITY ____________________ STATE __________ ZIP__________

PHONE (HOME) ______________ PHONE (WORK) ______________

TODAY'S DATE ______________ BIRTH DATE ______________

MARITAL STATUS __________

CHILDREN:

NAME AGE MAJOR HEALTH PROBLEMS

____

____

____

____

____

IS YOUR FATHER ALIVE? ____ IF NOT, WHAT WAS THE CAUSE OF DEATH?

____

____

DOES HE OR DID HE HAVE ANY OTHER MAJOR HEALTH PROBLEMS? DESCRIBE.

____

____

IS YOUR MOTHER ALIVE? ____ IF NOT, WHAT WAS THE CAUSE OF DEATH?

____

____

____

____

DOES SHE OR DID SHE HAVE ANY OTHER MAJOR HEALTH PROBLEMS? DESCRIBE.

____

____

BROTHERS AND SISTERS:

NAME AGE MAJOR HEALTH PROBLEMS

____

____

____

____

DO YOU FEEL CLOSE TO YOUR FAMILY?

____

____

WHAT IS YOUR OCCUPATION? ____________________________________

WHAT DO YOU DO WHEN YOU'RE NOT AT WORK?

____

____

WHY ARE YOU DOING "BEE-ACUPUNCTURE?"

____

____

____

____

HOW LONG HAVE YOU HAD THIS PROBLEM?

____

____

WHAT HAVE YOU DONE ABOUT IT?

____

____

____

____

WHAT WOULD YOUR LIFE BE LIKE IF YOU DIDN'T HAVE THIS PROBLEM?

____

____

____

____

IS THERE ANYTHING ELSE IMPORTANT THAT YOU WANT TO MENTION OR ANYTHING ELSE YOU NEED HELP WITH?

MEDICAL HISTORY:

CHILDHOOD ILLNESSES:

MAJOR/SERIOUS ILLNESSES:

PHYSICAL OR EMOTIONAL TRAUMAS:

SURGERIES/HOSPITALIZATIONS:

OTHER MEMORIES THAT STAND OUT:

WHAT ARE YOUR NORMAL SLEEPING HOURS? ______________________

DO YOU SLEEP WELL? ____ DO YOU WAKE UP AT NIGHT? IF SO, WHEN?

____

WHAT DO YOU DREAM ABOUT?

____

____

HOW IS YOUR APPETITE?

____

____

WHAT IS YOUR DIET LIKE?

____

____

WHAT KINDS OF FLUIDS DO YOU DRINK?

____

____

DO YOU DRINK ALCOHOL? IF SO, HOW MUCH?

____

____

ARE YOUR BOWELS REGULAR?

____

____

DO YOU HAVE DIFFICULTY WITH URINATION? ______________________

DO YOU PERSPIRE NORMALLY? ______________________________

DO YOU EVER GET COLD HANDS AND COLD FEET? __________________

DO YOU FEEL YOUR SEXUAL ENERGY IS HIGH, LOW OR NORMAL?

____

FOR WOMEN ONLY:

HOW OLD WERE YOU WHEN YOU FIRST STARTED YOUR PERIOD? __________

HAVE YOU EXPERIENCED PAIN, CRAMPING, BLOATING OR MOOD SWINGS?

____

____

METHOD OF CONTRACEPTION (IF ANY)? ______________________

HAVE YOU EVER SMOKED? DO YOU NOW? ______________________

ARE YOU TAKING ANY MEDICATION? IF SO, WHAT KIND? ______________

____

HAVE YOU EVER HAD HEPATITIS? ______________________

AS FAR AS YOU KNOW, HAVE YOU BEEN EXPOSED TO THE AIDS VIRUS?________

____

WHAT IS YOUR FAVORITE SEASON? ______________________

WHAT IS YOUR WORST SEASON? ______________________

WHAT IS YOUR FAVORITE TIME OF DAY? (BE SPECIFIC) ______________

WHAT IS YOUR WORST TIME OF DAY? (BE SPECIFIC) ______________

DO YOU HAVE SYMPTOMS AT THE SAME TIME EVERY DAY? IF SO, WHAT ARE THEY?

____

____

WHAT IS YOUR FAVORITE CLIMATE? ______________________

WHAT IS YOUR WORST CLIMATE? ______________________

WHICH DO YOU PREFER: HUMIDITY OR DRYNESS? ______________

WHAT IS YOUR FAVORITE COLOR? ______________________

WHAT IS YOUR WORST COLOR? ______________________

WHAT IS YOUR FAVORITE TASTE: SOUR, BITTER, SWEET, SPICY, OR SALTY?

WHAT IS YOUR WORST TASTE?: SOUR, BITTER, SWEET, SPICY, OR SALTY?

IF YOU COULD WAVE A MAGIC WAND, WHAT DO YOU REALLY NEED RIGHT NOW?

____

____

WHICH OF THE FOLLOWING IS THE MOST IMPORTANT TO YOU?

BEING LOVED UNCONDITIONALLY ____

FEELING UNDERSTOOD ____

FEELING RESPECTED AND APPRECIATED ____

FEELING REASSURED THAT EVERYTHING IS GOING TO BE OK ____

HAVING A SENSE OF DIRECTION ____

AFTER READING THIS BOOK, I BELIEVE THAT I AM MOST OUT OF BALANCE ON THE FOLLOWING ELEMENT: CIRCLE ONE

WOOD FIRE EARTH METAL WATER

EXPLAIN WHY:

____

____

____

____

THE SECOND ELEMENT THAT IS OUT OF BALANCE FOR ME SEEMS TO BE:

WOOD FIRE EARTH METAL WATER

EXPLAIN WHY:

____

____

____

____

I HAD TROUBLE DECIDING WHICH ELEMENT WAS MOST OUT OF BALANCE, BECAUSE IT FEELS LIKE THEY ALL ARE OUT OF BALANCE: YES/NO

I THINK THAT I AM MOST OUT OF BALANCE ON THE FOLLOWING PATHWAY:

GALL BLADDER LIVER HEART SMALL INTESTINE

HEART PROTECTOR THREE HEATER STOMACH SPLEEN

LUNGS COLON BLADDER KIDNEY

EXPLAIN WHY:

____

____

____

____

I THINK I AM ALSO OUT OF BALANCE ON THE FOLLOWING PATHWAYS:

____

EXPLAIN WHY:

____

____

____

____

I HAVE NOTICED THE FOLLOWING RESULTS USING "BEE-ACUPUNCTURE:"

____

____

____

____

____

____

____

____

____

____

PLEASE SEND THIS FORM TO: AMBER ROSE
5419 ROOSEVELT STREET
BETHESDA, MARYLAND 20817

ALSO SEND ANECDOTES TO THE SAME ADDRESS
FOR A FUTURE COMPANION BOOK.

The Multi-Center Apitherapy Study (NMCAS)

Intake Form #1

(Note: to be filled in by patient PRIOR to first treatment)

PLEASE PRINT Date______________ Age________ Sex: M____ F____

Name____Phone# (   ) ______________

Address____

City: ____State________Zip___________

Name of your MD ____

Address:____

City____State:__________Zip___________

Doctor's Telephone # (   )____

Date Your Symptoms began________________ Date You were Diagnosed ______________

Medical Diagnosis____

Diagnostic Tests used ____

Symptoms (in detail!) ____

____

____

____

List all meds you have tried for this problem with their effects and their side effects.

1____

2____

3____

4____

5____

6____

7____

Do you have a bee sting kit? Yes ______ No ______
Have you been instructed in the risks and benefits of apitherapy? Yes _____ No ______
Does your doctor know about your use of apitherapy? Yes ____ No ______
How did you learn about apitherapy? ______________________________________

Return ASAP to: MCAS

P.O. BOX 54 HARTLAND FOUR CORNERS. VT 05049 PHONE: 800.823.3460 FAX: 802.436.2827

The Multi-Center Apitherapy Study

Hey, are you what you eat after all?...

Your current **vitamin** or **nutritional supplements** with dosages, purpose and duration.

1)

2)

3)

4)

5)

6)

7)

Check which of these you take. Zinc ____ Magnesium ____ Beta carotene ______ Vit C______

Vit E ____ Essential Fatty Acids (fish or flax seed oil etc.) ____ Vit A _____ Digestive enzymes _______

B vitamins: Thiamine (B1) _____ Riboflavin (B2)_____ Niacin (B3)_____ Pyridoxal HCL (B6)_______

Cobalamine (B12) _____ Pentothenic Acid_____ Other supplements ______________________

Bee pollen _____ Raw Honey _____ Propolis _____ Royal Jelly ______ Homeopathic meds __________

DIETARY HABITS (describe a typical day's food and drink).

Vegetarian? yes____ no ____ Number of glasses of water a day: ______

Breakfast:

Lunch:

Dinner:

Snacks:

TOXINS: (How much a day and how many days a week do you take these substances? If you are not currently using them, please note your past use.)

Beer /Wine/Liquor: Recreational drugs:

Tobacco: Colas: Caffeine: Sugar: Ice Cream:

Return ASAP to: MCAS

P.O. BOX 54 HARTLAND FOUR CORNERS. VT 05049 PHONE: 800.823.3460 FAX: 802.436.2827

Initial Intake Form for Apitherapy

NOTE: Fill this form out prior to treatment.

Name________________________________ Phone______________

Address____

Town______________________________ State________________

Zip______________ Your Age______ Your gender M______ F_____

Medical Diagnosis_______________________________________

Date Symptoms began__________ Physical/Emotional Symptoms______

____

____

List all meds you use or have used_________________________

____

Date BVT began_________ Who stung you_______________________

stings per visit __________ Total# to date _______________

NUTRITIONAL INFORMATION

How much of the following do you take? Vit C _______________

Riboflavin (Vit B2) ____________ Pyridoxine (Vit B6) _________

Pentothenic Acid ______________ VitE _______________________

Honey ___________ Pollen ___________ Tobacco ________pack/day

Coffee__________ cup/day Alcohol __________________________

RELEASE OF INFORMATION:

Please do_____ do not _____ keep this information confidential.

Your signature_______________________________ Date___________

Bee Venom Therapy follow-up

First Visit Date.................... Referred by...

Persons present..

....

Info given : BVT reactions : anaphylaxis.........generalized..........local..........generalized delayed...............................

Vit C 6 Gm.......Rx for anakit and info about its use..........Tested for allergy ....

Neurologist: Name..Phone #..................................

Position vis a vis BVT...

# of stings given.......Response to stings: local...

general...

Plans for continuation...

Support phone #...................................||..

Follow up (with Dates)..

....

....

....

....

....

....

....

....

....

....

....

....

....

....

....

....

....

....

....

....

....

....

....

....

....

....

....

....

Th. Cherbuliez, M. D. printed on: 94.03.13

BEE STING ADVERSE REACTION

Reporter: Name ______________________________ Date ______________

Address ____

Phone # (____) ______________________________

Person Stung: Name (Optional) ______________________________

Age ____________ Diagnosis (if any) ______________________________

Circumstances of the sting: First time stung? Y/N ________

For demonstration? Y/N ________

For treatment? Y/N ________

If not first time, then earlier stinging history:

Approximately how many stings already received?__________ For what period of time? ______________

Any previous reactions? (describe) ______________________________

____

Current Incident: Date and time of the sting ______________ Time and date when reaction began ______________

Measures taken and outcome: ______________________________

____

____

____

To mail or fax to: **Th. Cherbuliez, M.D.**
1209 Post Road
Scarsdale, NY 10583-2023 **Phone/Fax (914) 723-0920**

AMERICAN APITHERAPY SOCIETY, INC.

Membership Application:

Note: if you are a current member who has not yet paid this year's dues, please renew now!

Name: ______________________ Title: __________

Address: ______________________ City: __________

State: __________ Zip Code: __________ Country: __________

Daytime Phone: __________ Evening Phone: __________ FAX: __________

Social Security Number ______________ **(Required for IRS exemption). Remember: AAS is a non-profit, tax-exempt corporation. The EIN is 16-1675818; Corp Tax Number is 0100-4352-57.**

MEMBERSHIP DUES:

I wish to become a:

_____ Member @ $35
_____ Donor @ $50
_____ Sustainer @ $100
_____ Patron @ $250
_____ Sponsor @ $500
_____ Benefactor @ $1000+

CONTRIBUTIONS:

I wish to contribute $__________ to the American Apitherapy Society.

PRODUCTS:

_____ copies of Annotated Bibliography of Apitherapy (specify Bee Venom, Raw Honey, Propolis, Royal Jelly, Wax, or Pollen) @ **$10 each.**
_____ copies of the 1977-1985 Apiotherapy Society proceedings @ **$25 each.**
_____ copies of Apitherapy Society Intro Packet @ **$5 each.**
_____ copies of *Bees Don't Get Arthritis* @ **$13 each.**
_____ copies of video: *Physician, Heal Thyself*, the Charles Mraz story @ **$50.**
_____ copies of video: *AAS 1993 Tour of China* @ **$50 each.**
_____ copies of AAS Membership List (avail. to members only) @ 10 **each.**

TOTAL (please make check to "AAS") ______________

Occupation and/or specialty: ______________________

Please tell us if you are a:

Apitherapist ______ Beekeeper ______ Apitherapy Patient ______ Illness ______________

Would you be available to answer questions from potential apitherapy patients, who want to learn about your experience using bee sting therapy? Yes _____ No _____

Will you accept referrals from people seeking treatment ideas? Yes _____ No _____

Do you want your name/address in the membership directory <u>for members only</u>? Yes _____ No _____

Today's Date ________ Your Signature (permission for us to publish your name) ______________

Please list names, addresses, and phone numbers of others whom you think might be interested in apitherapy.

1. ______________________ 2. ______________________

Please make your check payable to "American Apitherapy Society". Donations are tax-deductible and greatly appreciated. They help us serve the flood of requests for information from people seeking better health through apitherapy.

We thank you!

(Please offer any suggestions on how we can improve our service to you!)

P.O. BOX 54 HARTLAND FOUR CORNERS, VT 05049 PHONE: 800.823.3460 FAX: 802.436.2827

APPENDIX V

HOPE STINGS ETERNAL

Reprinted with Permission from

The Washington Post

CAN BEE VENOM HELP MS PATIENTS?

by Ken Ringle

Pat Wagner's house looks much like any other suburban rancher in the Waldorf neighborhood of Pinefield—apple tree in the front yard, two-car garage and, on the kitchen window, stickers with slogans like "Grandmothers Are Special and Start Each Day With a Song."

But if you watch awhile you might notice the two beehives in the back yard, and you'd certainly note the traffic coming and going—crippled people in wheelchairs and electric carts, unsteady people with canes and walkers, wasted, twisted figures carried in and out through the extra-wide door—all looking to get stung.

Most of those entering and leaving suffer from multiple sclerosis, the most degenerative nerve disease for which there is no known cure, and for them 5431 Lucy Lane in Charles County has become a place of cautious hope.

From 11 a.m. to 2 p.m. each Monday, Wednesday and Friday, Wagner and an ever-shifting handful of volunteer assistants treat the lethargy, numbness and paralysis of a growing number of MS sufferers with bee stings. She needs no medical license because she asks for no fee and promises no cure, but the zeal of a missionary among the tribes of the heathen, she urges those who seek her out to believe in an infant science called apitherapy. And under her hands—and as she insists, the hands of anyone attentive to the few known precepts of bee venom healing—some of the lame are walking, the numb are feeling and the physically drained say they're finding new life.

John Richert, a neurologist and the director of the Multiple Sclerosis Center at Georgetown University Hospital, says there is no scientific proof that bee stings benefit

MS patients. "But while you have to be skeptical you can't just dismiss the anecdotal evidence that there's more to all this," he says.

"No one's ever done the sort of large double-blind study you need to evaluate something like this," he says.

Meanwhile, listen to Perry Holmes Jr., a 38-year-old Fort Washington real estate broker diagnosed with MS four years ago who, after four bee sting sessions with Wagner, reports increased strength in his legs, improved sense of balance and an enormous increase in his daily energy level.

"I'm not going to get my hopes up yet about the long-term benefits," he said last week, waving a still-unsteady hand at the two dozen people crowding Wagner's kitchen and living room, "but I promise you, something is happening in here. We can't all be crazy."

Part of the difficulty in evaluating any treatment for MS lies in the unpredictable course of the disease. It has no known cause and rarely affects any two people in exactly the same way. It usually strikes gradually (numbness in the feet is a frequent first symptom) and, as it progresses, inhibits any of a number of motor skills. But it can just as easily disappear entirely for months or years, or reduce a healthy person to a permanently frozen skeleton in a matter of months.

"Sometimes people show extremely dramatic improvements, for no clear reason, just as we're ready to give up on them," says Richert. "In fact, it's not at all clear that MS is just one disease. The symptoms we associate with MS may be the product of several diseases, one of which may respond to one kind of treatment while another does not."

Pat Wagner, 42, is her own best advertisement for bee stings. She was diagnosed in 1970 with chronic progressive MS, the most serious variety, and within four years she retired on disability from her job as a program assistant for the U.S. Department of Labor.

Over the next two decades she experienced recurring and increasingly severe periods of numbers in her legs, weakness in her arms and torso, muscle spasms, blurred vision, impaired hearing and balance, bladder and bowel incontinence and severe lethargy. By early last year, she was totally wheelchair-bound, couldn't read or even feed herself. Doctors told her there was little hope of improvement. Kristy Hickey, who lives just across the street, remembers attending a wedding where Wagner was so weak and helpless she had to be carried in.

But Last year a friend of the family who had heard about apitherapy told Wagner about it and on March 24, 1992, she had herself stung for the first time. "When there's no hope, you try anything," Wagner explains.

A friend of a friend brought over some bees in a jar, she remembers. "He came into my bedroom—you have to realize none of us knew anything about how to do this then—and took out a bee and had it sting me on the inside of my left knee."

If you have MS, Wagner says, "your legs feel frozen . . . like ice water's running through your veins. But within 20 minutes it felt like warm blood was flowing down my leg. My whole leg began to get warm. I couldn't believe it. Then I took four or five more stings on my legs and three on the top of my body and soon my whole body felt warm. It was like this surge of energy through my veins. I no longer felt exhausted."

She was still largely immobilized and continued to suffer from blurred vision, she says. But after two months of additional stings, administered in a comparably haphazard fashion, "my hearing was totally back and I was out of the wheelchair and walking with a cane."

Even more significant, she says, was her sense of renewed energy and empowerment. "I had been taking all this medication, yet I was exhausted all the time, and so depressed I'd cry at the drop of a hat. Now I felt I could do anything."

Today, though still troubled with minor vision problems and occasional uncertain balance, Wagner is a virtual whirlwind, organizing seminars on apitherapy, handing out literature, phoning up television stations to spread the word and turning her home into a free clinic.

She has knocked out a wall in her house to accommodate the crowds of wheelchairs, printed up bee-bearing business cards ("Ask the Bee Lady about Honey

Bee Therapy") and has written articles for the quarterly newsletter of the American Apitherapy Society, BeeWell.

"When you touch somebody's arm or leg and they feel nothing, that bothers me," she says, "I know what that's like. I can't stand it and I want to help."

Stuart Goodman, Wagner's neurologist at Southern Maryland Hospital in Clinton, confirms Wagner's description of her condition last year. But he says it's not unusual for an MS patient in that condition to improve so dramatically, bee stings or no bee stings. And what's least clear of all, he says, is whether the improvement is physical—i.e., organic—and permanent or merely symptomatic and temporary.

"For example," he says, "I have a number of MS patients now who've been taking bee sting treatments. I'm not sure any of them have actually repaired their nerve damage. But all of them say they feel better."

The Kitchen Clinic

It's a little before noon on a typical sting day on Lucy Lane, and the atmosphere in Wagner's house lies somewhere between a faith-healing session and a Tupperware party. Some two dozen people mill around inside, crowding all the way to the family room mantelpiece that holds the dance trophies of Wagner's daughter Jessica, a 1982 princess in the Waldorf Turkey Bowl.

At The kitchen table, under a ceiling-hung stuffed bee and next to an apitherapy license plate ("Bee All That You Can Bee"), Pat Wagner sits questioning her patients, teasing them, calling greetings and being cheerleader as much as therapist. On the crowded table beside her sits a large Breckenridge Farms Mix Nuts jar, holes in its blue plastic lid, in which several dozen bees can be seen feeding on honey-soaked tissue and buzzing against the sides.

From time to time Wagner lifts the lid and sprays the bees with water from a plant mister "to quiet them and make them easier to catch."

After learning the specific complaint of each patient and his previous dosage (patients work up to as many as 20 stings per session) she opens the jar, extracts a bee with a pair of long-handled tweezers and applies its abdominal stinger to a bared part of the patient's body, then drops the dying bee into an empty mustard jar.

"Here comes a bladder sting (for incontinence). You're gonna love this," she tells a woman from Vienna, VA. "Just roll down the top of your panties. Just the top now! Everybody's watching and you're gonna be on 'Candid Camera.' Just tell your husband you got your BS degree at TSU. That's your bee sting at Ten-Second University."

The woman wants to be stung at home next time so she won't have the two-hour commute to Southern Maryland, so Wagner calls to her husband, Ray ("We call him 'Sting Ray'"), "Honey, we need a jar of bees to go!"

This is the fourth session for the Vienna woman, who says she's noticed no real improvement in her own troubled balance and uncertain walking, but has noticed improvement in others. "If you've got MS you grasp at straws," she says. "What do we have to lose?"

Wagner's visitors range from a Chilean economist retired from the Organization of American States to a tattooed firefighter with the Silver Hill Fire Department. The latter administers the test stings—antidote kit at the ready—on all first-time patients to test their allergic reaction before any treatment starts.

Some patients keep records for Wagner, others hand around liability waivers and literature. Treatment is roughly first-come, first-served, but if someone has a special need others willingly step aside.

"Those people in there are so warm and so caring it's unbelievable," says Reginald Herron, echoing the volunteered remarks of almost all of Wagner's visitors. Herron, 35, lives off Martin Luther King Boulevard in Southeast Washington and had brought his father for his first treatment. "It's like a big family for everybody in there . . . really beautiful."

Nobody, he says, asked him for money or even mentioned it. He had to ask the whereabouts of the small honey jar marked "Hive $" where donations can be left. Wagner says her highest weekly take so far is $65.

One of those getting stung is Ed McIver, 45, a wheelchair-using allergist, retired on disability, who was diagnosed with MS during his first year in Howard Medical School. He receives 14 stings in this, his third session, most of them in the back of his neck. Since starting such treatment three weeks ago he's noticed "a significant increase in energy," much easier breathing and speech, plus some additional mobility in his left hand, which he says was curled into a claw before and has somewhat straightened out.

"It's hard to know why this works," he says. "Emotions play so heavy a part in this disease it could be just the support group here . . . knowing someone who has the disease is getting better. It's so easy to be depressed with a disease that has no cure."

But in addition, he says, "the stings seem to stimulate the immune system and there is some indication the bee venom forces the adrenal gland to produce steroids. Steroids are one thing used to treat MS, often with some success."

It also helps, he says, "to believe in acupuncture. If you notice where she's stinging people, it's basically in the same trigger points they use for acupuncture."

Perhaps the worst case on hand is that of Irene Phelps, 46, of Upper Marlboro, whose thin body is curled in a wheelchair and who talks only with difficulty. She's suffered from chronic progressive MS for 11 years and has come for her sixth session, taking 20 stings.

Before treatment started, she says, she couldn't even straighten her legs. Now her body is much more relaxed and she's less tired.

"It gives you a little hope. Doctors give you no hope at all," says her husband, John, 55, a semi-retired contractor. Like most of those in the Wagner house, the Phelpses learned of Wagner and apitherapy from a local television news show last fall, "and it looked like something natural that we should try," John Phelps says. I'm a country boy and I know there is a lot of natural things we've forgotten that are better than what any doctor can do."

The Beekeeper's Discovery

Apitherapy probably started with the first bee, but most of its formal history in this country appears to lead back to a Middlebury, Vt., beekeeper named Charles

Mraz. Mraz, now 88, says he's been "fooling with bees since I was 14, and all the old-timers then used to tell me bee stings were good for arthritis. And of course, being 14, I thought they were crazy."

Then, when he was 28, he was stricken with rheumatic fever, which left him not only heart-damaged but with pain in his joints so severe "I couldn't get out of a chair." After suffering for six months, "I remembered what those old guys had said and decided what the hell and took a couple of bees and stung myself on either side of one knee. I woke up the next morning and the pain was entirely gone. And that was quite a shock."

In the years since, Mraz has talked up his treatment to doctors, and offered it free to anybody suffering from rheumatic diseases. Then, in 1986, he says, a woman came to him with MS. "I told her didn't know anything about MS. She said, 'Well, you treated me for arthritis five years ago and the symptoms went away. When they came back I went to a doctor and he said they were really due to MS. So you were really treating MS last time and it worked. Treat me again.'"

Three years later he formed the American Apitherapy Society together with Bradford Weeks, a physician in general practice in North Hartford, Vt. Weeks says his role has been to "provide the scientific documentation for the extraordinary work done by Charles Mraz. People come from all over the world to be treated by him, but he keeps no records. Nor does he charge them. As he always says, he's not a doctor, he's just a beekeeper. So I started keeping records for him. We now have a computer database with about 6,000 patients on it, more than 300 of them with MS."

Their efforts, he says, have triggered extraordinary research interest in places like France and Korea, where he says he and Mraz have been flown in to lecture, and where major government scientific studies are underway. "But until recently there's been no corporate or government money available for major controlled studies in this country. The potential corporate profits just aren't there."

According to Georgetown Hospital's Richert, the most intriguing aspect of bee venom is a compound in it called apamin. The symptoms associated with multiple sclerosis, he points out, result from the inflammatory degeneration of the nerve sheaths that carry electrical signals to and from the brain. "When a sheath degenerates, it doesn't conduct electricity very well, so the nerve impulses get blocked. Apamin doesn't stop the degeneration, but it improves the conductivity of the degenerated sheath. That may very well be what's at work in the MS cases where bee venom has shown success."

In addition, Weeks says, the venom contains two extraordinarily powerful anti-inflammatory agents, melittin and adolapin, which appear to fight the neural sheath inflammation itself.

Richert, however, says bee venom is merely the latest in a succession of natural substances touted as promising cures for MS in recent years. Cobra venom, for awhile, was another.

He himself has tracked four patients being treated with bee venom therapy, none of whom, he says has shown any long-term improvement.

Yet "there's more than a little evidence that beekeepers as a group are unusually healthy and long-lived, and may have unusual immune systems. Maybe bee stings have something to do with that. We have a grant application in to fund a major double-blind study on bee venom, where neither the patient nor the physician knows who's getting the tested drug and who's getting the placebo. That's the only way to prove a treatment's effectiveness."

Meanwhile, Weeks says the immune-stimulating properties of bee venom have prompted its use in the treatment of other diseases such as lupus, asthma and inevitably, AIDS.

It's only an experimental treatment for AIDS, he says. No one is calling it a potential cure. "We have 10 people with AIDS being treated with bee venom now," Weeks says. "The results are very, very preliminary. The biggest problem is that people with AIDS are taking so many drugs simultaneously it's almost impossible to say for sure which one is causing any beneficial effect. But there are some promising signs."

Anecdotal Evidence

Back at Pat Wagner's, Jane Terry is explaining how MS affects the social life of a modern young woman in Georgetown. "The biggest problem," she signs, "is leaving puddles. If I could cure anything it would be the incredible weakness in my left leg and foot so when I know I have to, I could run to the john in time."

Terry, a wide-eyed 26, makes MS sound a bit like an unfair parking ticket—really annoying, but, like, what are you gonna do?

She was diagnosed with MS during her junior year at Mount Vernon College, and has tried "every therapy around . . . . Nothing did much. I was so lethargic it was all I could do to take my dog out. I was pathetic!"

But since beginning bee stings three weeks ago, she says, she's had "this huge rush of energy. I run around now all over the place. And though I still leave puddles occasionally—this is really gross and embarrassing but you can't imagine how you treasure small victories—I haven't wet the bed! For the first time since I had MS!"

Today she's had more bladder stings plus a number of stings on her left leg. As she's explaining how things could really be much worse, she suddenly stops and makes a startled "Oh!"

"I just crossed my legs!" she says.

It's true, she did.

"But you don't understand," she says. "I haven't done that for two years. And look at this!"

She holds up her left leg and rotates her foot. The ankle is red and throbbing, covered with bee stings, painful-looking as an open wound. But Terry is smiling it's Christmas.

"Isn't that a hoot?" she says.

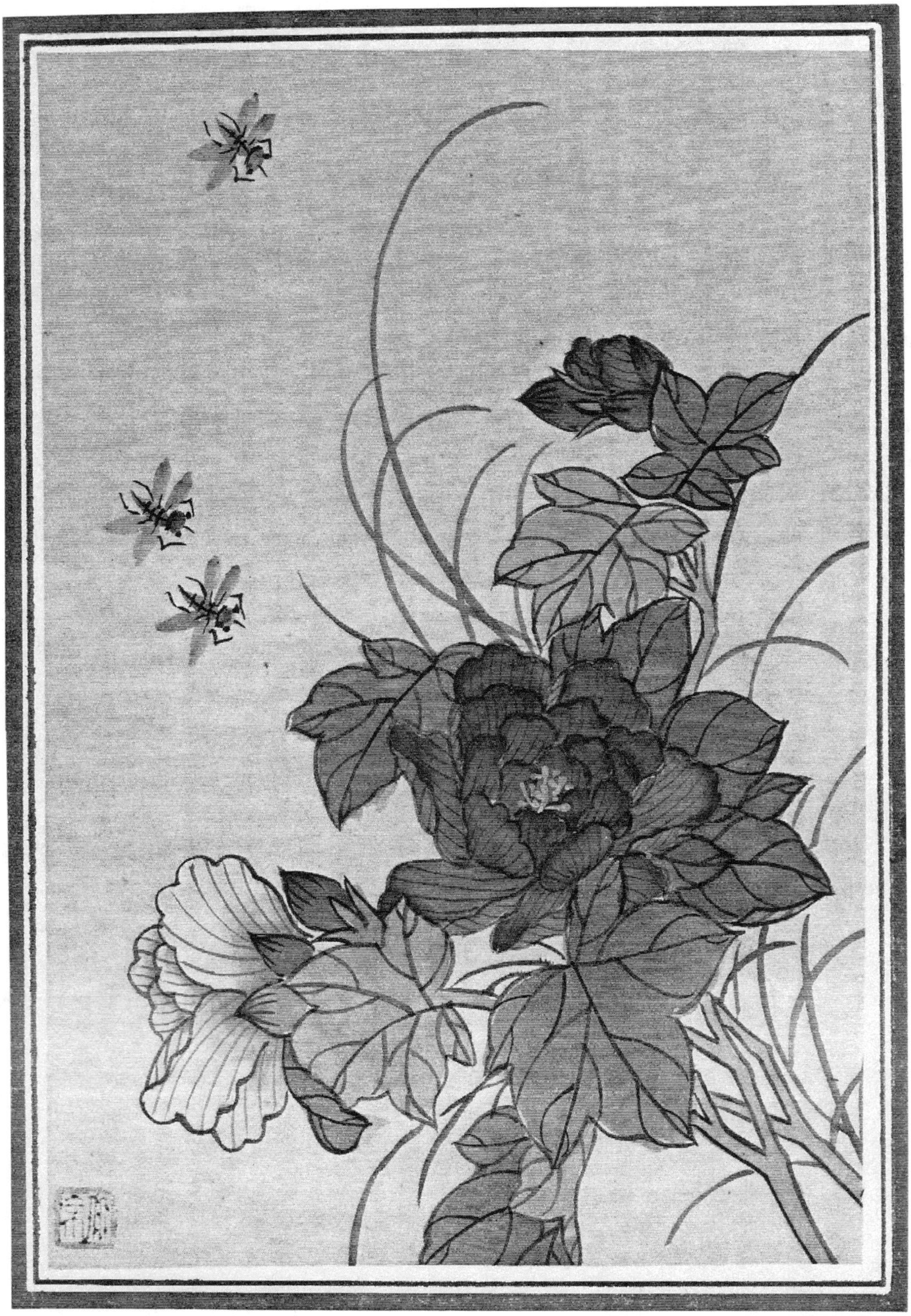